Risk Management
BASICS

*Protecting Profits and Product Safety in
Medical Product Industries Through Risk-Based
Decision-Making in Change Control, Deviation Investigations,
and Corrective/Preventive Action Programs*

**Carol DeSain
Charmaine Vercimak Sutton**

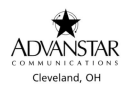

Cleveland, OH

DEDICATION: TO "US"!

Copyright © 2000 Advanstar Communications Inc.

All rights reserved. No portion of this book may be reproduced or used in any form or by any means—graphic, electronic, or mechanical, including photocopying, recording, taping, or information storage and retrieval systems—without written permission of the publisher.

Printed in the United States of America

10 9 8 7 6 5 4 3 2 1

ISBN 0-929870-55-7

Library of Congress Catalog Card Number 00-106392

Published by Advanstar Communications Inc.

Advanstar Communications is a worldwide business information company that publishes magazines, directories, books, produces expositions and conferences, provides a wide range of marketing services, and maintains numerous Websites.

For additional information on any Advanstar product or for a complete catalog of published books, please write to: Advanstar Customer Service, 131 West 1st Street, Duluth, Minnesota, 55802 USA; or visit www.advanstar.com.

To purchase additional copies of *Risk Management Basics*, please call 1-800-598-6008; outside the U.S. call 218-723-9180. Order on-line at www.boreal.org/tamarack/books.html.

Publisher/Product Manager: Danell M. Durica
Cover and Interior Design: Dave Crouch Graphics. Cleveland, Ohio

Contents

INTRODUCTION 1

SECTION I – DETERMINING RISK FOR PRODUCTS AND PROCESSES DURING DEVELOPMENT

CHAPTER 1: PRODUCT RISK ANALYSIS 7
Risk Analysis in the Product Lifecycle 8
Performing Product Risk Analysis 8
Severity and Probability Rankings 10
Risk Level Matrix 10
Product Hazard Identification and Severity Ranking Assignment 12
Cause Identification and Probability Ranking Assignment 13
Overall Risk Assignment 15
The Product Risk Analysis Report 16
Routine Use of the Risk Analysis Report 16
    Risk minimization during product development 16
    Risk-based decision making during routine operations 17
    Risk-based decisions when product and
    process changes are proposed 17
Keeping the Risk Analysis Report Current 18
Retrospective Risk Analysis 18
Product and Process Risks 19

Exhibit 1.1 Product Risk Analysis Report 21
Exhibit 1.2 Phase II: Bottom-Up Risk Analysis Table 22

CHAPTER 2: PROCESS HAZARD ANALYSIS AND CRITICAL CONTROL POINT IDENTIFICATION **25**
HACCP 26
Process Control Points vs. Critical Control Points 27
Performing Process Hazard Analysis and
Critical Control Point Identification 27
    Critical process identification 27
    Critical process hazard analysis and
    critical control point determination 28
    Support process hazard analysis and CCP identification 29
    Process flow hazard analysis and CCP identification 29
Essential Control Points: An Opportunity 29
Control Point Limits 30
Process Validation 30
Identification of CCPs and ECPs in Routine Processing 30
Exhibit 2.1 Process Control Point Evaluation Record 31

SECTION II – RISK MANAGEMENT SYSTEM BASICS

CHAPTER 3: RISK-BASED DECISION MAKING FOR INFORMATION MONITORING PROGRAMS IN OPERATIONS **35**
Types of Information Monitoring Programs 37
Monitoring Control Standards:
Distinguishing Data-of-Compliance
from Data-of-Exception Observations 38
Data-of-Exception Observations:
Preliminary Investigation Requirements 39
    Confirmation 39
    Triage 40
    Preliminary investigation records and notification 41
Information Monitoring Program Development 41
    Normal operating conditions, alert limits,
    action limits, and specifications 43
Information Monitoring Program Implementation,
Training, and Data Entry Management 43

Data-of-Compliance Trending 44
Exhibit 3.1   Out-of-Specification Result Observation
              and Preliminary Investigation Record 45
Exhibit 3.2   Environmental Monitoring
              Program Document Example 47

CHAPTER 4: RISK-BASED DECISION MAKING FOR POST-MARKET FEEDBACK INFORMATION MONITORING PROGRAMS 51

Monitoring Programs for Post-Market Feedback Information 52
    Complaint monitoring for adverse events 52
Preliminary Evaluation of Complaints 54
    Complaint review and information gathering 54
    Complaint triage 55
    Decision trees 57
    Preliminary evaluation records and notification 57
Action Implementation 57
Actions Taken Before Investigations Are Complete 57
Trending Data-of-Exception and Data-of-Compliance Observations . . .58
Actions Taken in the Market 58
Risk Analysis Updates with Post-Market Information 59
Exhibit 4.1   Decision Record: Data-of-Exception
              Observations from Post-Market Feedback Information . . .61

CHAPTER 5: RISK-BASED DECISION MAKING IN FORMAL INVESTIGATION, ACTION IDENTIFICATION, AND AUTHORIZATION 63

Formal Investigation Criteria 64
Formal Investigation Teams 64
Formal Investigation Team Meetings 65
The Formal Investigation Process 66
    Phase 1 – Investigation initiation and problem definition 66
    Phase 2 – Gathering of information for problem characterization 67
    Phase 3 – Determine and verify cause 68
    Phase 4 – Action analysis and action authorization 70
    Phase 5 – Action implementation and follow-up 71
Exhibit 5.1   Information Gathering for
              Investigations in Operations 74
Exhibit 5.2   Formal Investigation Record 75
Exhibit 5.3   Action Review Record 78
Exhibit 5.4   Regulatory Review Record 79

CHAPTER 6: RISK-BASED DECISION MAKING IN ACTION IMPLEMENTATION AND EFFECTIVENESS ASSESSMENTS 81
Action Planning 82
   Direct action implementation 82
   Action implementation planning 83
   Action tracking records, logs, and notifications 83
When Action Is Required Before the Investigation Is Complete 84
Actions Required by Regulatory Authorities for Distributed Products ...84
Exhibit 6.1   Action Implementation Planning Protocol 86

SECTION III – MANAGING FOR SAFETY AND PROFIT

CHAPTER 7: WHY THINGS GO WRONG: ACCIDENT THEORIES IN INNOVATIVE/ TECHNOLOGICALLY COMPLEX INDUSTRIES 89
Types of Accidents 90
Accident Theories 92
High Reliability Theory Perspective on Organizations 93
Normal Accident Theory Perspective on Organizations 94
High Reliability vs. Normal Accidents 95
Accidents-of-Management 96
   Normalization of deviance 96
   Information reporting variables 97
   Summit fever 98
   Crisis and stress 99
Management Is Responsible for the Decision-Making Environment 99

CHAPTER 8: MANAGING RISK-BASED, DECISION-MAKING GROUPS TO PROTECT PROFITS AND PRODUCT SAFETY 101
Segregation of Technical Risk-Based Decision Makers
from Business Risk-Based Decision Makers 102
   Symptoms of business culture dominance 103
Risk-Based Decision-Making Group Organization,
Performance, Training, and Monitoring 104
   Establish a clear, focused mission for the group 104
   Establish work input, work flow,
   work conduct, and output criteria 105
   Train and develop risk-based decision-making groups 105

Integrate information between risk-based decision-making groups . .106
Monitor and control of group performance 107
Decision-Making Meeting Controls 109
Agenda consistency 109
Meeting notification and preparation requirements 110
Information quality, analysis, and presentation requirements 110
Rules of conduct 111
Rules for decision-making 111
Group leadership 112
Leadership from Management 112
Be an advocate for risk-based decision-making 112
Accept conflict and confrontation as essential to
risk-based decision-making 113
Avoid cultures of blame 113
Know when to seize authority and when to let go 114
Consider the cultural influences beyond the corporation 115
Provide confidence and optimism 115
Stay connected 115
Monitor group performance 115
When management fails 117
The extra challenges of innovative technologies 117

**CHAPTER 9: ORGANIZATIONAL DESIGN:
A NEW APPROACH** **119**
A New Organizational "Chart" 120
People-Based vs. Function-Based Organizational Designs 122
Establish Functional Units-of-Operation for the Organization 123
Establish Roles and Responsibilities for
Functional Units-of-Operation 124
Designate Authority and Responsibility 125
Managing the Responsible Worker 125
Exhibit 9.1   Business Units, Quality System
             Components, and Functional Units-of-Operation 127
Exhibit 9.2   Quality System Component
             Documents: Format and Content Guidelines 130
Exhibit 9.3   Example Quality System Component Document 131
Exhibit 9.4   Example Quality System Component Document 134

GLOSSARY **137**

INDEX **145**

FIGURES

Figure 1.1 – Product Risk Analysis Events 9
Figure 3.1 – Risk Management Framework 36
Figure 9.1 – Organizational Design
             That Supports Risk Management 121

Introduction

Business success is assured when innovative, problem-free products are created to fulfill a customer's greatest expectations affordably and at a profit to the company. Investors support companies that are quick to market new products; workers are dedicated in companies that maintain stress-free working environments; customers are loyal to brands that have worked for them before; and regulators reward companies that manage their problems effectively and efficiently with quicker access to markets and less oversight. **Enthusiastic investors, dedicated workers, loyal customers, and friendly investigators are not discovered, they are created.**

"Build a quality product and they will buy" has been the mantra of the quality revolution. Quality, however, comes in degrees and costs money. Determining how much quality is enough becomes the challenge of business executives. The VP of Quality may argue for quality at any cost, but the VP of Marketing knows that the product will have significant market competition if product launch is delayed past September.

How much quality is enough? It depends on the product, the patient population, the user group, and the industry, but every company *must* design and manufacture safe products that perform as intended. Safety and performance standards, determined by corporations and regulators, are achieved when there are no serious accidents associated with product use. The degree of quality assurance required, therefore, is the amount necessary to prevent accidents without compromising a product's ability to meet its intended use or the company's ability to make a profit.

Accident theories developed from high-technology, innovative industries (Chapter 7) provide insight into the challenge of balancing profit and product safety in the medical product industry. Studies from high-technology industries (nuclear power generation and aviation) suggest that successful risk management in medical product development/manufacturing is closer than may be imagined. After all, the tools of risk analysis, change control, investigation, and corrective/preventive actions have already been established in response to regulatory expectations. The industry has not, however, learned to manage these tools effectively. In the absence of effective and efficient management, there is never enough quality, there is never enough investigation, there is never enough information, and there is never enough money.

Three types of accidents have been identified: accidents of design, accidents of procedure, and accidents of management. (1, 2)

Accidents of design are material, process, and product failures that should be predicted and eliminated, or prevented during product/process design and validation, but are not. For example:

- "An American Eagle ATR turboprop dives into a frozen field in Roselawn, Indiana, because its de-icing boots did not protect its wings from freezing rain . . . and as a result, new boots are designed."
- "A USAir Boeing 737 crashes near Pittsburgh because of a rare hard-over rudder movement . . . and as a result, a redesigned rudder-control mechanism is installed in the whole fleet."
- "A TWA Boeing 747 blows apart off New York because, whatever the source of ignition, its nearly empty center tank contained an explosive mixture of fuel and air . . . and as a result, explosive mixtures may in the future be avoided." (1)

Accidents of procedure are accidents that occur because mistakes occurred during product use. When pilots fly into violent thunderstorms, which is not accepted procedure, accidents are likely to occur. If pilots fly airplanes in icing conditions, without undergoing a de-icing procedure, accidents are likely to occur.(1) These are not accidents of design, they are accidents of procedure.

As the medical products industry learns to develop products and their associated manufacturing processes in a controlled manner, potential accidents of design and accidents of procedure will be eliminated and/or their impact will be minimized *before* the product is available for commercial use. This is accomplished by:

- identifying hazards associated with the product design/use or process design/use,

- determining the risk that these hazards pose to product safety/performance,
- eliminating high-risk hazards or minimizing the impact of high-risk hazards through re-design, when possible,
- identifying remaining product/process risks in a manner that enables Commercial Operations to make risk-based decisions about product/process deviations and changes that maintain an appropriate balance of profit and product safety.

These elements of risk management, however, require a framework for product development, routine operations, and commercial distribution that is anchored in the product safety imperatives of the market. In this text, the anchor of risk management is presented in Section I and the risk management framework is presented in Section II.

- Section I identifies the systematic processes of hazard identification, risk analysis, and risk reduction procedures used in Product Development and Validation to identify product and process risks in a manner that facilitates their use in Commercial Operations.
- Section II identifies the systematic processes of information monitoring, deviation triage, problem investigation, action planning, action implementation, and action effectiveness assessments used in Operations, Quality Assurance, and Customer Service to identify, correct, and/or prevent accidents of design and accidents of procedure in the market.
- Section III discusses why establishing the processes described in Sections I and II are not enough to ensure risk-free product use and performance. Accidents of management, which can have as great an impact on product safety as accidents of design and accidents of procedure, are presented.

At the root of all accidents-of-management is the fact that product safety requirements compete for the same resources that keep products affordable and corporations profitable. As a result, when management decisions about resource allocation are not aligned with product risk analysis, these decisions are vulnerable to both production pressures (favoring corporate profit over product safety) and extraordinary QA/Regulatory expectations (favoring product safety over corporate profit). Management decisions create the relationship between profit and safety, and established patterns or bias in management decision making will be maintained by the workforce. When the relationship between safety and profit is not properly balanced by management, the health of the patient and/or the company is compromised consistently. Once a risk management framework is established, as suggested in this text, management can prevent or control accidents-of-design, accidents-of-procedure, and accidents-of-management, and keep the corporation well balanced between profitability and providing medical benefit to their markets.

CITED REFERENCES:

1) Langewiesche, William. 1998."The Lessons of Valu-Jet 592." *Atlantic Monthly* (March).

2) Sagan, Scott D. 1993. *Limits of Safety*. Princeton, NJ: Princeton University Press.

SECTION I

Determining Risk for Products and Processes During Development

CHAPTER 1

PRODUCT RISK ANALYSIS

Product risk analysis forms the backbone of risk-based decision-making processes in a medical product company. Product risk analysis identifies all potential hazards posed by product use to the patient and/or product user, and categorizes those hazards according to severity and probability of occurrence. Two benefits of product risk analysis are that accidents can be mitigated and important decisions in product development and commercial manufacturing can be based on product risk.

Accidents are mitigated when the risk analysis report identifies specific unacceptable risks posed by the product and then a planned program for risk mitigation is defined and implemented during product development. In the end there will be documented evidence that all reasonable efforts were taken to reduce known product risks to acceptable levels, and residual risks associated with the product will be clearly identified.

TABLE 1.1: RISK ANALYSIS TERMINOLOGY (1)

Risk analysis	the use of available information to identify hazards and estimate risk.
Hazard	a potential source of harm.
Harm	physical injury and/or damage to the health of people, property, or the environment.
Risk	the combination of the probability of occurrence of harm and the severity of that harm.
Severity	a measure of the possible consequences of a hazard.
Residual risk	risks remaining after protective measures have been taken.

Product risk analysis also provides a basis for making important decisions in product development, commercial manufacturing, and the market. When the costly decisions associated with verification testing, process validation, deviation investigations, and corrective/preventive actions are product focused, the safety of the patient is protected with an efficient use of corporate resources. The use of product risk analysis and process hazard analysis (Chapter 2) in a product-focused quality system is presented in Section II of this book.

RISK ANALYSIS IN THE PRODUCT LIFE CYCLE

As shown in Figure 1.1, product risk analysis forms the backbone on which all other product-associated activities are grounded during the life cycle of the product. Product risk analysis is performed and a report is created initially during product development when final product specifications are first drafted. The Product Risk Analysis Report is then consulted during the following activities:
- planning process development
- conducting manufacturing process hazard identification
- planning/designing process validation studies
- planning/designing product qualification and validation studies
- collecting information about product and process performance
- investigating deviations and out-of-specification (OOS) results during commercial operations
- making preventive/corrective action planning decisions during commercial operations
- updating products and improving their safety and usefulness.

Using a Product Risk Analysis Report to support decision making throughout the product life cycle will provide consistency in the decisions made under pressure by groups of people with variable alliances to the product. Without established, predetermined decision-making criteria, different groups of people are likely to draw different conclusions for perfectly good reasons. For example, if components fail QC testing at a time when Production is desperate for parts, Production is likely to reconsider whether the failure is all that important. If the component was assigned a 'critical' designation by a group of experts at an earlier time, however, and this predetermined judgment must be consulted during routine decision making, Production is less likely to make a poor decision under pressure.

PERFORMING PRODUCT RISK ANALYSIS

There are many standards, guidelines, and resources for analyzing product risks (see References at the end of this chapter). Most of these standards have the following common elements:

FIGURE 1.1: PRODUCT RISK ANALYSIS EVENTS

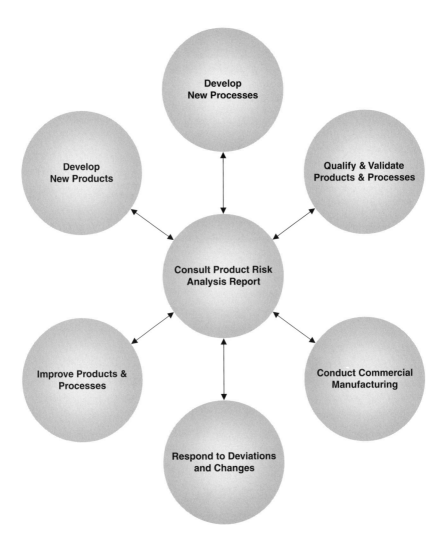

- severity and probability rankings
- a risk level matrix that distinguishes acceptable risks from unacceptable risks by relating the severity of an effect-of-failure to the probability that the failure will occur
- product hazard identification and severity ranking assignment
- cause identification and probability ranking assignment
- an overall assignment of a risk level for each identified hazard.

SEVERITY AND PROBABILITY RANKINGS

Although any risk analysis process is dependent upon severity and probability rankings, there are no industry-accepted standards for severity and probability rankings and no standard for combining those rankings to define risk levels. As a first step in the product risk analysis process, therefore, each medical product developer/manufacturer must define his or her own product-specific severity and probability rankings.

Severity rankings are used during the product risk analysis to indicate the anticipated extent of harm caused by a particular product feature.

TABLE 1.2: SEVERITY RANKING EXAMPLES

Abbreviation	Severity Ranking	
CA	Catastrophic	High potential for patient death
CR	Critical	High potential for serious injury
M	Marginal	Clinical complications not listed as CA or CR
N	Negligible	Minor clinical effect, not likely to result in any complication

Probability rankings are used during the product risk analysis to indicate the expected frequency of occurrence of a hazard presented by a particular product feature.

TABLE 1.3: PROBABILITY RANKING EXAMPLES

Abbreviation	Probability of Ranking	
F	Frequent	Greater than 1 in 10
O	Occasional	Between 1 in 1,000 and 1 in 100
R	Remote	Between 1 in 10,000 and 1 in 1,000
IM	Improbable	Between 1 in 100,000 and 1 in 10,000
IN	Incredible	Less than 1 in 100,000

RISK LEVEL MATRIX

Hazard probability and severity rankings are combined in a matrix to determine risk levels. Again, there is no industry-accepted standard for risk level determination, and each medical product developer/manufacturer must develop their own. In the example provided below, three risk levels are identified: acceptable (A), unacceptable (U), and acceptable with justification (J). The "J" category is used when there is a risk that cannot be minimized beyond current design and product users appear to accept the risk when balanced with product benefit. In the example matrix below, the severity rankings are placed on the x-axis, the probability rankings on the y-axis, resulting in 24 spaces in which to place U's, J's, and A's.

TABLE 1.4: RISK LEVEL MATRIX

		N	M	CR	CA
PROBABILITY	F	J	U	U	U
	P	J	U	U	U
	O	A	J	J	U
	R	A	J	J	U
	IM	A	A	J	U
	IN	A	A	J	J
		SEVERITY			

U = Unacceptable risk
J = Acceptable risk with justification
A = Generally acceptable risk

As an example, the following criteria were used to place the risk levels in the matrix:
- All catastrophic severity hazards were assigned U for unacceptable, except for catastrophic severity hazards having an "incredible" probability of occurrence, which were assigned J.
- All frequent and probable hazards were assigned U for unacceptable, except for frequent and probable hazards with a negligible severity, which were assigned J.
- No critical severity hazards were assigned A for generally acceptable risk.
- Negligible severity hazards were assigned A for generally acceptable risk, except for negligible severity hazards with high (frequent or probable) probability, which were assigned J.
- Marginal severity hazards that were highly unlikely to occur (improbable or incredible probability) were assigned A for generally acceptable.

Risk level assignments may change during the product development process, based on new information from, for example, clinical investigations and published reports of commercial use of similar products. Risk level assignments may also change based on market experience.

Product Hazard Identification and Severity Ranking Assignment

When the severity and probability rankings and the risk level matrix have been created, the actual product risk analysis can begin. Product risk analysis is performed in two phases. The first phase is a top-down risk analysis, representing the perspective of the user (e.g., physician, consumer/patient, equipment operator). The second phase is a bottom-up risk analysis, representing the perspective of the product design or formulation. Both phases of risk analysis, which represent two approaches to hazard identification, are useful at different points in product development and manufacturing, for different reasons. Together they provide a complete risk analysis.

The top-down phase of the product risk analysis is performed by a multifunctional team comprising representatives from Regulatory, Clinical, Marketing, Manufacturing, Quality, and Product Development. A table such as the one in the Product Risk Analysis Report in Exhibit 1.1 should be used to facilitate the risk analysis and capture the results.

In the top-down risk analysis:
- each stage of product use is identified beginning with the user reading the product label and deciding whether to use the product and ending with the user discarding the used product.
- all potential final product failure modes and the possible adverse user effects of those failures are identified for each stage of product use.
- a severity code based on the established severity categories is assigned to each possible adverse effect.

Top-down hazard identification asks, "From the perspective of the user and user environment, what could go wrong with the product in its entire life cycle, from the time it is shipped to when it is discarded?" If the User Requirements have been previously documented, a top-down hazard identification can be facilitated by referring to the User Requirements document and asking, "How can the product fail to meet the User Requirements and subsequently pose harm to the user?" When User Requirements have not been determined previously by Product Development, develop a list of user expectations, identify all adverse effects that could occur if the user expectation is not met, and assign a severity ranking to each adverse effect.

Product:
- blood-contact catheter product sealed in sterile barrier

User Requirements/Expectations:
- sterile barrier packaging is intact (undamaged) upon opening.
- product is biocompatible.

- product does not fall apart under (what the user considers to be) normal conditions of use.

Possible adverse effects:
- infection caused by microbiological contamination
- toxic response to catheter materials
- embolism of a catheter part that separates during use

Severity rankings for the adverse effects:
- infection – critical
- toxic response – critical
- embolism – critical

The purpose of this analysis is to identify and categorize all significant potential clinical effects or hazards for the user, patient, or environment. It is best, therefore, to perform this phase of risk analysis early in the product development process so that risk minimization (safety) can be designed into the product. This top-down phase is not a stand-alone risk analysis, however, because the phase ends when the hazards have been identified and categorized and does not extend the analysis into determining the probability of occurrence and risk level assignments.

CAUSE IDENTIFICATION AND PROBABILITY RANKING ASSIGNMENT

In the second phase of product risk analysis, the bottom-up approach, possible failure modes for product components, subassemblies or process intermediates, and final product are identified and linked to the potential hazards already identified in the top-down phase. The likely causes of each failure mode are then identified, along with any known failure-mitigating factors. Finally, a probability that the failure will occur and lead to the hazard is assigned to each failure mode.

The bottom-up product risk analysis is typically led by a representative from Product Development and performed with appropriate input from Clinical/Field Support, Manufacturing, Regulatory, and QA representatives. A table such as the example in Exhibit 1.2 at the end of this chapter is prepared to facilitate the analysis and capture the results.

Bottom-up hazard identification asks, "What could go wrong if a particular product component or subassembly fails?" and "What is the probability that it will fail?" During the bottom-up product risk analysis:
- all potential failure modes associated with a particular component, subassembly, or final product feature are identified;

- the failure modes are linked to a potential user adverse effect identified during the top-down risk analysis;
- possible causes for each failure mode are identified, along with mitigating factors; and
- a Probability is assigned to each cause of failure, based on the established probability rankings and later on results from product verification and validation studies.

For example:

Product specification:
- a final assembly drawing that identifies catheter shaft materials, bond strengths, and a sterility assurance level for the packaged, sterile product

Potential failure modes:
- product not sterile
- material not adequately specified
- inadequate bond strength

Potential user effects (from top-down risk analysis):
- infection – critical
- toxic response – critical
- embolism – critical

Failure mode causes:
- inadequate sterile barrier seal, inadequate sterile barrier material
- nonbiocompatible catheter materials
- weak tip-to-shaft bond

Failure-mitigating factors:
- industry standard materials and sealing equipment; validated sealing process; qualified package design
- biocompatibility test results; confirmation that material specification accurately reflects the material tested
- bond strength verification testing that shows only a moderate level of confidence or reliability

Probability of occurrence (with mitigating factors considered):
- sterile barrier seal or material fails, goes undetected, results in non-sterile product being used, leads to infection — improbable
- wrong material is used to make product, goes undetected, results in patient exposure and toxic response — improbable
- weak bond goes undetected, fails during use, results in embolism – probable

The assignment of probability rankings can be started at any time; it cannot be completed, however, until information about probability of occurrence is available (e.g., data from design verification and validation studies).

The bottom-up approach ensures a more comprehensive and detailed review of the product for possible failure modes than the top-down approach. This approach cannot be used until there are specifications for components, formulations, intermediates, and subassemblies. The bottom-up approach should be performed when specifications are first drafted, after product verification and validation studies are complete, and when significant changes to the components, formulations, or intermediates are proposed.

OVERALL RISK ASSIGNMENT

Based on the Severity and Probability ranking assignments, and using the Risk Level Matrix, a residual risk—e.g., either generally acceptable, acceptable with justification, or unacceptable—is determined for each cause of failure. Any risk judged unacceptable must be reduced to an acceptable level before beginning commercial production and/or marketing the product.

Risk Level Assignments:
- inadequate sterile barrier seal, inadequate sterile barrier material
  - Probability — improbable
  - Severity of potential effect (infection) — critical
  - Risk Level Assignment — J (acceptable with justification)
- nonbiocompatible catheter materials
  - Probability — Improbable
  - Severity of potential effect (toxic response) — critical
  - Risk Level Assignment — J (acceptable with justification)
- weak tip-to-shaft bond
  - Probability — probable
  - Severity of potential effect (infection) — Critical
  - Risk Level Assignment — U (unacceptable)

Plans can now be made to reduce risks identified as 'unacceptable' to an acceptable level before releasing the product to commercial production. For example, design verification testing may have demonstrated that a safety-critical bond between the catheter tip and shaft failed often enough to be considered an unacceptable risk. The bond must be improved, therefore, to reduce the frequency of failure to an acceptable level before the product is released to commercial production.

Planned product verification or validation testing may be indicated in the risk analysis tables by inserting a protocol identification number or "protocol to-be-determined" and identifying the department responsible for completing the work. When the planned studies are completed, the relevant report number(s) may be recorded in the risk analysis report and the probability of a failure occurring and risk level are updated as indicated by the study results.

THE PRODUCT RISK ANALYSIS REPORT

When a product risk analysis has been completed, the information should be summarized in a Product Risk Analysis Report. The Report is a controlled document approved by representatives from the participating departments, e.g., Regulatory, Clinical, Marketing, Manufacturing, Quality, and Product Development. It should contain:

- name, model, and current revision or part number of the product analyzed
- category definitions, i.e., Severity, Probability, or Risk Level or reference to these definitions in other controlled documents
- risk analysis tables, such as the examples in Exhibits 1.1 and 1.2
- change history logs, forms, or tables that provide a detailed description of changes to the Product Risk Analysis Report and rationale for changes made to the report after its initial issue.

ROUTINE USE OF THE RISK ANALYSIS REPORT

The product risk analysis report should not just be filed away as evidence that a regulatory requirement was met. It should be used routinely to:

- guide risk minimization efforts during product development
- make risk-based decisions during routine operations and in response to post-market feedback
- make risk-based plans for qualifying product changes.

RISK MINIMIZATION DURING PRODUCT DEVELOPMENT

Risk minimization, or risk control, must be undertaken for any risk that was determined to be unacceptable as a result of the product risk analysis. The risk minimization effort should be focused on:

- eliminating or reducing the risk by inherent safe design or redesign
- reducing the risk by protective measures
- reducing the risk by providing adequate user information and sufficient warnings.

If the risk cannot be reduced by one of these measures, then a risk-benefit analysis should be performed and documented in the product risk analysis report. The risk-benefit analysis should be based on objective data and literature on the efficacy of the product, and should contain a clear conclusion about whether the medical benefits outweigh the risk.

When new risk control measures are introduced into the product, including new warnings or precautions in the labeling, the effectiveness of those measures should be verified. A focused product risk analysis should then be performed to demonstrate that the new measures have in fact reduced the risk level, and to assess for new hazards presented by implementing the new controls.

Risk-based decision making during routine operations

The Product Risk Analysis Report should be consulted when important decisions are made about deviations, changes, and actions taken during routine operations. Risk-based decision making in routine operations can reduce the cost of compliance. Risk-based decision making provides benefit to decisions about:

- process validation and revalidation requirements
- the rigor of sampling, inspection, and testing of materials
- the rigor of inspection, testing, and/or sampling of process parameters, processing intermediates, processing environments, and processing equipment
- material or process change qualification requirements
- the seriousness of deviations from procedure and out-of-specification results (Chapter 3)
- the seriousness of product complaints (Chapter 4)
- the adequacy of proposed corrective and/or preventive actions (Chapter 6).

Risk-based decisions when product and process changes are proposed

When significant product or process changes are proposed, the Product Risk Analysis Report should be consulted to help decide how much change qualification work should be done before the change is implemented. If the product feature that is the subject of the change is not listed in the risk analysis report, then risks associated with the proposed change should be analyzed and incorporated.

When change is proposed, refer to the Product Risk Analysis Report and identify the severity rankings assigned to the hazards associated with the relevant product feature. If the highest Severity ranking is:

- Negligible or Marginal — then the change may be handled through established action implementation procedures, e.g., Direct Action Implementation in Chapter 6.
- Critical or Catastrophic, and the change results in the addition or deletion of one or more final product specifications — then the change

requires development of a modified product according to established Product Development procedures, e.g., Design Control procedures (21 CFR 820.30) for device and diagnostic products.
- Critical or Catastrophic, but the change does not add or delete final product specifications — then the change may be handled by performing a planned product verification or validation study to confirm continued compliance with existing specifications, and then handled through established action implementation procedures, e.g., Direct Action Implementation in Chapter 6.

A new risk analysis is expected when any of the following occur:
- the feature is not listed because the proposed change contributes a new feature;
- the feature is not listed because the change involves a feature that was previously overlooked; or
- the change of one feature could affect a previous judgment of risk for another feature.

KEEPING THE RISK ANALYSIS REPORT CURRENT

To ensure consistent application of the severity and probability categories, the risk analysis report should be maintained by a trained expert. The Product Risk Analysis Report should be reviewed and revised as needed when product changes are proposed, and when substantial new safety and/or performance/effectiveness data is collected, such as:
- data from formal clinical investigations
- data from post-market surveillance/complaint handling programs
- reports of unanticipated adverse events.

Keep a detailed history of change for the Product Risk Analysis Report that identifies the versions of the report generated over time, an associated version number, the date of issue, changes made to the report and the rationale/justification for change, and reference to any supporting information or studies that support the change.

RETROSPECTIVE RISK ANALYSIS

Retrospective risk analysis is performed for products already in commercial distribution, when product risk analysis has not been conducted previously. Retrospective product risk analysis, like prospective risk analysis, is used to support deviations and changes to a product and its associated processes over time. The primary difference between conducting a prospective and a retrospective product risk analysis is that a retrospective analysis relies on existing information about product risks. Information about product hazards and their severity and frequency (probability of occurrence) should be available in clinical investigation reports, customer complaint reports, and public reports of product safety and performance. Similarly, information about the probability of occurrence of some product failure modes should be available from product testing records.

A retrospective product risk analysis begins with an information-gathering phase to collect any documents that may contain information about the safety and performance of the product or product family. In all other aspects, a retrospective product risk analysis is performed in essentially the same manner as a prospective product risk analysis. The ability to use documented product safety and performance information may reduce the need to have product development and clinical research experts on the product risk analysis team, but the process remains the same.

PRODUCT AND PROCESS RISKS

Performing a product risk analysis is essential when designing safe products that minimize the risk and likelihood that accidents-of-design and accidents-of-procedure will occur with routine product use. There are some hazards, however, that can be introduced into products with variability in raw materials, manufacturing processes, testing processes, critical processing environments, and processing equipment. The hazards of processing, therefore, also need to be identified and controlled as presented in Chapter 2.

CITED REFERENCES

1. ISO 14971: Medical Devices — Application of risk management to medical devices.
2. Military Standard: Procedures for Performing a Failure Mode, Effects and Criticality Analysis MIL-STD-1629A, 1980.

REFERENCES

"Analysis Techniques for System Reliability: Procedures for Failure Mode and Effects Analysis (FMEA)." IEC 60812.

"Analysis Techniques for System Reliability: Procedures for Fault Tree Analysis (FTA)." IEC 1025.

MIL-Std-882C. 1993. "System Safety Program Requirements." Philadelphia: Naval Publications and Forms Center.

Modarres, M. 1993. *What Every Engineer Should Know about Reliability and Risk Analysis.* New York: Marcel Dekker.

European Commission. 1998. "Medical Devices: Risk Analysis." (EN 1441) Brussels, Belgium.

Stamatis, D. H. 1995. *FMEA from Theory to Execution*. Milwaukee, WI: ASQC Quality Press.

United Kingdom. Ministry of Defence. 1989. "Requirements for the Analysis of Safety Critical Hazards" (draft). May.

United Kingdom. Ministry of Defence. 1991. "Hazard Analysis and Safety Classification of the Computer and Programmable Electronic System Elements of Defence Equipment. *Interim Defence Standard 00-56*. 5 April 1991.

U.S. Department of Commerce. Technology Administration, National Institute of Standards and Technology Computer Systems Laboratory (NISTIR 5589). "A Study on Hazard Analysis in High Integrity Software Standards and Guidelines," by L. M. Ippolito and D. R. Wallace. 1995

Exhibit 1.1

Product Risk Analysis Report
PHASE I: TOP-DOWN RISK ANALYSIS TABLE
Product: Tofte Catheter Model 55615

Page __1__ of __1__

Report ID# _____   Version _____

Associated Product Specification Number: PS_____   Rev. _____

Product status: ( ) pre-design verification/validation   ( ) commercially available product change
                 ( ) post-design verification/validation

CLINICAL EFFECTS LIBRARY for Tofte Catheter
(select and use only effects from the following list)
- Pain
- Infection, possibly requiring antibiotics and prolonged hospitalization
- Fever
- Problem is detected before or during product use and product is discarded with no clinical effect
- Damage possibly requiring surgical repair or other intervention
- Distal emboli possibly requiring percutaneous or surgical intervention
- Toxic reaction
- Allergic reaction
- Transmission of viruses

SEVERITY CATEGORIES

Severity Ranking		Qualification
CA	Catastrophic	High potential for patient death
CR	Critical	Serious injury, need for surgical repair
M	Marginal	Clinical complications not listed as CR or CA
N	Negligible	Minor clinical effect, just noticed, not likely to result in any complication

1	2	3	4
item #	Potential final product failure modes	Potential adverse effect of the failure	Severity
1.			
2.			
3.			
4.			
5.			
6.			

( ) See attached meeting minutes and supporting documentation.
( ) Change history updated.

TOP-DOWN RISK ANALYSIS REPORT APPROVALS:

Product Development _____ Date _____   Clinical Research _____ Date _____

Quality Assurance _____ Date _____

EXHIBIT 1.2

Product Risk Analysis Report
PHASE II: BOTTOM-UP RISK ANALYSIS TABLE
Product: Tofte Catheter Model 55615

Page 1 of 2

PROBABILITY* Rankings

Abbreviation	Probability of Occurrence	
F	Frequent	Greater than 1 in 10
O	Occasional	Between 1 in 1,000 and 1 in 100
R	Remote	Between 1 in 10,000 and 1 in 1,000
IM	Improbable	Between 1 in 100,000 and 1 in 10,000
IN	Incredible	Less than 1 in 100,000

*Probability that, despite the mitigating factors, the cause will occur *and* lead to the failure mode *and* result in the clinical effect.

Risk Level Matrix

PROBABILITY	N	M	CR	CA
F	J	U	U	U
P	J	U	U	U
O	A	J	J	U
R	A	J	J	U
IM	A	A	J	U
IN	A	A	J	J

SEVERITY

U = Unacceptable risk
J = Acceptable risk with justification
A = Generally acceptable risk

Exhibit 1.2 (continued)

Product Risk Analysis Report
PHASE II: BOTTOM-UP RISK ANALYSIS TABLE

Page __2__ of __2__

#	1 Product Feature (reference specification ID# or drawing ID#)	3 Potential Failure Mode	4 Potential Adverse Effect of Failure[1]	5 Severity of Clinical Effect[1]	6 Cause of Failure	7 Mitigating Factors +/- Revelant Product Verification & Validation Report #	8 Risk Analysis Result (after V & V) Prob / Risk	9 Planned Action + Responsibility (shaded if no actions are planned)
1.								
2.								
3.								
4.								
5.								

( ) See attached meeting minutes and supporting documentation.
( ) Change history updated.

BOTTOM-UP RISK ANALYSIS REPORT APPROVALS:

Product Development _____ Date _____ Quality Assurance _____ Date _____

[1] from top-down risk analysis report

CHAPTER 2

PROCESS HAZARD ANALYSIS AND CRITICAL CONTROL POINT IDENTIFICATION

As a product is developed, manufacturing processes are identified that will create or isolate the proposed product; and test methods are identified that will provide evidence that the manufacturing processes, in fact, produce acceptable product. Once identified, product manufacturing and testing processes are validated to demonstrate that they will perform reliably and consistently in the manufacturing and testing environment. Once validated, they are monitored to assure consistent performance and to detect unexpected change during routine use.

In this scenario processes are systematically developed and transferred to the user environment, and process validation is considered sufficient to assure that potential accidents-of-design (resulting from poorly designed processes) and potential accidents-of-procedure (resulting from misuse of these processes by technicians or line workers) have been adequately eliminated or their impact minimized *before* they are authorized for use in the commercial product manufacturing/testing environment.

Although process validation has improved process development and process transfer, it has resulted in excessive validation commitments and excessive process monitoring requirements for routine manufacturing. Increased information about processes, however, has not improved process reliability. In spite of good process validation studies and vigilant process monitoring, it remains difficult to know how to react responsibly when process controls fail to meet established limits or acceptance criteria.

It is difficult to react responsibly to process deviations because responsible decision making requires, in addition to validation, a predetermined evaluation of process hazards and their potential connection to product hazards. Process validation as currently practiced does not provide adequate benchmarking for the continuing evaluation of process deviations throughout the process life cycle. As a result, when a process control limit is not met for a validated process during routine production, is the process considered ineffective? It depends. It depends on what the process is designed to do; it depends on the impact that loss-of-control has on the product; and without predetermined analysis of hazards, it can depend on who conducts the investigation.

Process hazard analysis, like process validation, is conducted to prevent and/or minimize the impact of accidents-of-design and accidents-of-procedure. In addition, process hazard analysis provides an opportunity to categorize process control points (PCPs) into levels-of-concern based on the impact that loss-of-control poses to product safety and performance. Predetermined categorization of PCPs facilitates a risk-based triage of process deviations throughout the life cycle of the process and provides an opportunity to balance the quality (safety) objectives of the corporation with its production (profit) objectives.

HACCP

The Hazard Analysis and Critical Control Point Principles and Application Guidelines (HACCP) developed in 1997 by the U.S. FDA, Department of Agriculture, and the National Advisory Committee on Microbiological Criteria for Foods provide a format for process control point identification and evaluation. The approach is similar to that provided in FDA's design control regulations for products, 21 CFR 820.30, as well as in international standards ISO 9001 and ISO 13485. The guideline was created to help food processors and distributors ensure that foods are safe for consumption by providing an "effective and rational means of assuring food safety from harvest to consumption. HACCP plans are narrow in scope, being limited to ensuring that food is safe to consume." (1)

The seven principles of HACCP are:
(1) conduct a hazard analysis
(2) determine critical control points
(3) establish critical control point limits
(4) establish monitoring procedures
(5) establish corrective actions
(6) establish action verification procedures
(7) establish record-keeping and documentation procedures

The only principles of HACCP that are not already components of existing quality systems in medical product development and manufacturing companies are principle #1: conducting a hazard analysis of processes, and principle #2: determining critical control points in processes.

PROCESS CONTROL POINTS VS. CRITICAL CONTROL POINTS

Process control points (PCPs) are the steps in processing where biological, chemical, or physical factors are controlled to provide greater assurance that a process will perform reliably. Some process controls are more important than other process controls, however, because failure-of-control at these process steps affects the safety of the product. These control points are called critical control points (CCPs). CCPs are distinguished from PCPs based on the type of hazards that they are designed to control, and as a result process hazard analysis is required to segregate CCPs from PCPs.

PERFORMING PROCESS HAZARD ANALYSIS AND CRITICAL CONTROL POINT IDENTIFICATION

Identification of CCPs is facilitated by conducting a hazard analysis of:
- critical processes
- support processes that support critical processing
- inter-dependent sets of processes.

CRITICAL PROCESS IDENTIFICATION

For each product, develop a list of all product manufacturing processes, test methods, and their associated documents, e.g., manufacturing or testing SOPs, Production Batch Records, Manufacturing Travelers, or Device History Records (Exhibit 2.1). Develop a flow diagram of the product manufacturing and testing processes, by document ID#, that identifies the following:
- the order of processing
- the interrelationship between processes
- the location of processing (manufacturing/testing site location and/or location of processing lines within the facility)
- any considerations for manufacturing cycles or campaigns based on the scale of manufacturing, pooling of intermediates, sublots, etc.

Identify critical product features by reviewing the product risk analysis report, if available, and/or by identifying all product features and performance requirements listed in the final product specification and labeling. Product features are designated as critical if lack of this feature or variation in its control would adversely affect product safety for the patient or the customer/user.

Finally, link each manufacturing and testing process to final product features. Every manufacturing process and the associated test methods should either create or support a final product feature or attribute. A filter sterilization process, for example, creates or supports the sterility attribute for that product; formulation and filling processes create and support the potency and uniformity characteristics of a product; labeling supports product dosage or usage requirements, etc. When this list is complete, critical processes are identified as those processes and test methods that create or support critical product features or attributes.

In sterile product manufacturing, for example, the depyrogentation process would be identified as a critical process, because failure of this process could affect the safety of the product. Similarly, the endotoxin test method would be identified as a critical process. When a formal product risk analysis has been performed and documented (see Chapter 1) this task is completed by simply looking up the criticality of the product feature in the risk analysis report.

Critical process hazard analysis and critical control point determination

Process hazard analysis requires the identification of potential hazards associated with processing. Hazards are conditions that could cause unreliable or ineffective processing. To identify hazards, potential failure modes for each process are identified by asking "What could go wrong?" Process hazard identification must consider the impact that variability or differences in materials/components, equipment/utility systems, processing/testing environments, and storage conditions or holding times for materials or intermediates could have on process reliability and effectiveness. When process development is complete, process control points are identified and in-process testing requirements established in SOPs, Production Batch Records, or Device History Records. These documents establish the materials, equipment, and the processing environment required for effective, reliable processing.

Critical control points (CCPs) in critical processes are identified by listing the existing process control points and determining if variability, difference, or failure in any individual PCP could affect process reliability or effectiveness; if so, it is a CCP. Most PCPs in critical processes are CCPs because deviation from these process control limits is likely to affect product safety.

In a steam sterilization process of final product (a designated critical process), for example, process controls (PCPs) include:
- chamber temperature*
- steam quality
- chamber pressure

- equipment identification/cycle configuration/time*
- load identification/configuration*

For closed vial products, CCPs would include (*) controls. Chamber pressure is related directly to temperature, and steam quality for closed vial products is not as critical (see discussion later in this chapter).

Support process hazard analysis and CCP identification

Processes that support critical processes must also be analyzed for hazards and identification of CCPs. Sterility testing, for example, is a critical process. Sterility testing is supported by many other processes, such as growth promotion testing of media, steam sterilization of media and/or test equipment, cleaning/disinfection of sterility testing environment, etc. All processes that support critical processes should be evaluated for CCPs. Growth promotion testing of sterility test media, for example, would be a CCP, because failure of the media to support growth could lead to a false negative in product sterility testing.

Process flow hazard analysis and CCP identification

Additional hazards can be identified from process flow diagrams. These are the hazards that exist when the relationship between processing and/or testing events is either not established or changes. Hazards can be created when, for example, processing intermediates are held before further processing in conditions that promote bacterial growth. These hazards are usually associated with changes in production scale, changes in production contractors, etc. Similarly, hazards can be created when samples are stored before testing in conditions that contribute to their deterioration or production equipment sits too long before cleaning and disinfection procedures are performed. Review the manufacturing and testing process flow diagrams and campaign manufacturing requirements for production areas and equipment to identify additional hazards and associated CCPs.

Essential Control Points: An Opportunity

In complex processing, such as fermentation, protein purification, steam-in-place, clean-in-place, or viral inactivation procedures, two types of control points (PCPs and CCPs) are not always sufficient. There are many control points that, although not directly related to product safety, are nevertheless essential for process reliability and effectiveness. PCPs that are not CCPs but are essential to product performance or process performance — in that deviation from processing limits or acceptance criteria would seriously compromise the reliability or effectiveness of the process — are called essential control points (ECPs). ECPs are also identified during process hazard analysis.

Control Point Limits

All ECPs and CCPs must have associated control point limits that are established and validated. These limits establish a range of values considered acceptable as a measure of the effectiveness of process controls. During routine processing it is expected that in-process testing results will fall within established limits. If there is a deviation from these limits, it is considered a significant deviation such as a Level III observation in Chapters 3–6.

Process Validation

All critical processes must be validated. All processes that contain CCPs should be validated. All CCPs and ECPs should be monitored during routine processing to assure the effectiveness of control. Process validation extends process development into the environment of use and increases the assurance that any process variables introduced by the users in the user environment do not affect process performance or reliability. This exercise, if successful, further reduces the probability that accidents-of-design or accidents-of-procedure will occur. Identifying CCPs and ECPs before validation studies are conducted can provide an opportunity to establish meaningful study acceptance criteria. Nevertheless, identifying CCPs and ECPs after validation studies are conducted can still provide the opportunity to react responsibly to process deviations, as will be discussed in Section II.

Identification of CCPs and ECPs in Routine Processing

In order to react responsibly to process deviations that occur during routine processing and testing, CCPs and ECPs must be clearly identified for the worker and the auditor. Although listing these control points in validation documents is essential, validation documents are seldom available in routine operations. Develop documentation conventions that consistently highlight CCPs and ECPs, e.g., italicized or bold text, formatting in shaded boxes, etc. Develop associated procedures for revalidation criteria and investigation criteria based on these control point designations.

Cited References

1. U.S. Food and Drug Administration, U.S. Department of Agriculture, and National Advisory Committee on Microbiological Criteria for Foods. "Hazard Analysis and Critical Point Principles and Application Guidelines." August 14, 1997.

Exhibit 2.1

PROCESS CONTROL POINT EVALUATION RECORD

Page __1__ of __2__

Process description _____

Process is currently established in document _____ version _____

Process is used to ( ) test ( ) produce ( ) support the following products: _____

Is this process a critical process ( ) yes ( ) no   Provide rationale for CCP designation _____

Process creates or supports what product features/attributes? _____

Has this process been previously validated? ( ) no ( ) yes   see _____

Will this process be validated ( ) no ( ) yes

Identify processes that support this process _____   Identify document ID# _____

Process review by _____ Date _____

Verification _____ Date _____

EXHIBIT 2.1 (CONTINUED)

PROCESS CONTROL POINT EVALUATION RECORD

Page __2__ of __2__

#	Material or process parameter that is controlled	Method of control +/- method ID#	Process control limits or acceptance criteria	Does failure-of or deviation-in control of this material or step impact product safety? yes / no / maybe	Identify CCP ECP PCP	If control is achieved by a support processing event, identify the process
1						
2						
3						
4						
5						
6						

Completed by _____ Date _____ Verified by _____ Date _____

SECTION II

RISK MANAGEMENT SYSTEM BASICS

CHAPTER 3

RISK-BASED DECISION MAKING FOR INFORMATION MONITORING PROGRAMS IN OPERATIONS

Information monitoring programs are designed to "watch over" the organization by collecting and assessing information generated from ongoing activities for compliance with established standards of practice. Two types of observations/information/data are collected from the monitoring of ongoing manufacturing, testing, and distribution of products: data-of-exception and data-of-compliance observations (Figure 3.1).

Data-of-exception observations include information, observations, or data that does not meet established standards of practice. Standards of practice in the medical product industry are established in procedures, protocols, batch records, device history records, specifications, and equipment-controlling software. A data-of-exception observation is anything that is not within acceptable, normal operating conditions including deviations, out-of-specification results, discrepancies, nonconfirming units, alert limits, action limits, and invalid test results.

Data-of-compliance observations include information or data that does meet established standards of practice. This is the "good information" that is used to release product into the market, and this is the information that can also be used to predict and prevent problems.

Data-of-exception and data-of-compliance observations collected from the routine activities of the corporation are managed differently. A data-of-exception observation requires immediate response, because it could indicate

FIGURE 3.1
RISK MANAGEMENT FRAMEWORK

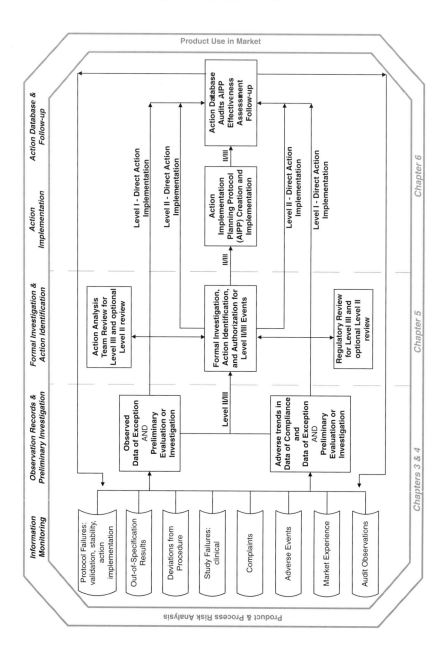

a problem that would seriously and adversely affect product safety or performance. Data-of-compliance observations require periodic review and trend analysis to detect potential problems.

Information monitoring programs must be established to collect data-of-exception and data-of-compliance observations within the organization and outside of it. Internal monitoring programs monitor the development, production, testing, packaging, labeling, and distribution of products. External monitoring programs monitor product use and product performance in the market and the user environment. Internal information monitoring programs will be discussed in this chapter; external programs are presented in Chapter 4.

Finally, information monitoring programs can benefit from a risk management framework (Figure 3.1) in which information monitoring and management practices are anchored to the Product Risk Analysis reports from Product Development. This integrated approach to risk management can improve the effectiveness and efficiency of troubleshooting, reduce the number of new or recurring problems, and reserve organizational resources for the most serious problems.

TYPES OF INFORMATION MONITORING PROGRAMS

Information monitoring programs are developed to assure that:
- products meet established specifications;
- product processing is compliant with expected performance standards;
- processing environments are compliant with expected standards;
- resources used to produce, test, and distribute products are acceptable; and
- quality systems are compliant with established procedures.

The number and types of information monitoring programs will be determined by the size and complexity of the organization. Some monitoring programs are software driven and information is collected electronically; some programs are manual and information is collected by line workers or technicians who make visual observations and create written records of the observations. Responsibility for monitoring should be retained in the functional area that is most knowledgeable about the product/process being observed. Monitoring for equipment performance in a water purification system, for example, should be performed by Maintenance; monitoring for water quality should be performed by Quality Control.

Consider the following list of information monitoring programs, common to medical product development and manufacturing environments:

Resource Quality Monitoring
Material Identity and Quality Monitoring
Equipment Monitoring: Preventive Maintenance, Calibration and Performance Monitoring
Environmental Control Monitoring: Bioburden, Temperature, Air Pressure Differentials, Humidity, Particulates, Electrostatic Discharge
Personnel Performance Monitoring

Process Performance Monitoring
Process Control Monitoring of Manufacturing Processes
Process Control Monitoring of Testing Processes

Product Monitoring
Product Release Testing/Monitoring Programs
Product Stability/Reliability Testing

Quality System Monitoring
Auditing of Manufacturing Areas
Vendor Certification
Client/Contract Review/Monitoring

Monitoring Control Standards: Distinguishing Data-of-Compliance from Data-of-Exception Observations

All observations derived from information monitoring programs must be recorded and compiled for further analysis. In addition, observations derived from monitoring programs must be judged, as collected, to be data-of-exception or data-of-compliance. Compliance or exception is judged from predetermined criteria established in controlled documents such as specifications, standard operating procedures, test methods, product batch records, or device history records. Every observation should be judged for compliance, as soon as possible after it has been recorded. Once judged, data-of-exception observations are managed on an event-by-event basis; data-of-compliance observations are reviewed periodically.

Design information monitoring programs to ensure that the information required to distinguish data-of-compliance from data-of-exception is readily available to the individuals likely to make the observations. This can be facilitated with data collection records designed both to collect and to judge the acceptability of the information as it is collected. Although this type of data collection and record-keeping requires a responsible workforce (see Chapter 9), because it asks more of the line worker than simple observation and documentation, the closer the judgment is in time to the observation, the more efficient the system.

DATA-OF-EXCEPTION OBSERVATIONS: PRELIMINARY INVESTIGATION REQUIREMENTS

Preliminary Investigations, sometimes referred to as informal investigations by regulators, must be conducted for every data-of-exception observation. The purpose of this investigation is to solve the simple problems and to initiate a risk-based triage on the remaining problems. The Preliminary Investigation takes place at the point of observation by the observer and/or a supervisor as soon as possible after the event has been recorded or observed. Preliminary Investigations should:

- confirm the data-of-exception observation
- perform a risk-based triage of the observation and assign a level-of-concern
- resolve most problems without the need for Formal Investigation by
  – identifying the cause of the problem, if readily apparent
  – recording actions and rationale for actions
- notify the Formal Investigation Team when further investigation is warranted.

CONFIRMATION

All data-of-exception observations must be confirmed by a second observer, usually a supervisor. The questioning that supports this review process should provide the first opportunity to characterize the problem, identify its cause, and take appropriate action. Consider the following review elements for observations made in the operating environment:

- Interview the individual who observed the deviation or problem about what he or she saw or heard, and what they think could be the problem.
- Review equipment performance and calibration records. Is there evidence of equipment failure? Review repair records, if appropriate. Look for obvious failure modes.
- Review reagent identification and performance. Ensure that the current version of the correct reagents were used within their assigned expiration dates. Is there any sign of reagent deterioration?
- Look for process or method deviations. Ensure that the current version of the correct procedure was used. Interview the observer about the procedure to ensure that it was followed. Indicate if this is the first use of a new procedure or a new version.
- Review calculations for errors, transposition of numbers, and missing information.

- Observe samples when appropriate. Are they completely and correctly identified? Indicate whether anything about the sample suggests that it was improperly handled.
- Assign a level-of-concern to the observation, as presented below. Consult any procedures associated with the observation for Critical or Essential Control Points (Chapter 2).

TRIAGE

Not all data-of-exception observations require the same rigor of investigation and analysis. Sorting these observations into "big deal" events and "little deal" events is necessary to ensure that the observation is relayed in a timely manner to the individuals most equipped to solve the problem. Triage is designed to assign priority to investigations, based on the perceived impact that the observation might have on the safety and performance of the product, the safety of the worker, the reliability of operations, market stability, or cost-effectiveness of operations. All data-of-exception observations are categorized into levels-of-concern based on an organization-wide, risk analysis for products (Chapter 1) and processes (Chapter 2).

Consider the following levels-of-concern:

Level III — This level contains data-of-exception observations that require *immediate* investigation and action. Level III observations must have potential impact on the safety of the product *and* the product must be in the market or the clinic, i.e., available for human use. Level III observations should be rare events. Candidates for Level III assignment include:
- stability study failures for commercial products stored at recommended storage conditions within labeled shelf-life
- out-of-specification results (OOSRs) associated with Critical Control Point limits (Chapter 2) for product already in distribution
- complaints or adverse events that involve serious injury or death are associated with product use, and are reportable (Chapter 4)
- observations classified as errors and accidents, as defined by 21 CFR 600.14
- observations classified as corrections and removals, as defined by 21 CFR 806
- observations classified as field alerts, as defined in 21 CFR 314.81.

Level II — This level contains data-of-exception observations that require Formal Investigation to determine cause and that require corrective or preventive action. Level II observations must have the potential to significantly affect product or process performance. Candidates for Level II assignment include the following:

- OOSRs for any product component or final product already in distribution
- OOSRs associated with Essential Control Point limits (Chapter 2)
- OOSRs associated with any stability study acceptance criteria for studies of product stored at recommended storage conditions within labeled shelf-life
- complaints or adverse events that do not involve serious injury or death

Level I — These are data-of-exception observations with a pre-defined response, such as a validated reprocessing event or a corrective action. Level I observations do not directly affect product quality. Level I assignments are appropriate when the cause is known and corrective action is obvious and easily implemented. Only Level I observations can be closed out at the department level at the completion of a Preliminary Investigation. Data-of-exception observation records should be designed to facilitate the close-out of all Level I observations by providing a record of the actions taken, and/or the rationale for not taking action. Consult Exhibit 3.1.

PRELIMINARY INVESTIGATION RECORDS AND NOTIFICATION

There must be a record of each Preliminary Investigation, indicating that it was conducted as directed. The record must be accompanied by any additional information gathered from the questioning, retesting, etc., to assist further investigation. Level I observation records should be submitted for entry into an action database as suggested in the Direct Action Implementation option in Chapter 6. Level II and Level III Observation/Preliminary Investigation Records (example provided in Exhibit 3.1) must be transferred to the Formal Investigation Team as soon as possible.

INFORMATION MONITORING PROGRAM DEVELOPMENT

Once a product, component, process, or environment is identified that requires monitoring to assure the effectiveness of control, an information monitoring program is developed. For example, when humidity levels in the manufacturing facility must be controlled to control static discharge, prevent bacterial growth, and minimize the rusting of stainless steel surfaces, one would develop a program that monitors humidity control by identifying the following:

1. The product, component, process, or environment to be controlled
   The manufacturing environment, specifically filling suite A

2. Control parameters, i.e., what will be controlled
   Humidity
3. Control mechanisms or procedures
   Humidity is controlled with steam piped into existing HVAC units; given the location of the facility in Arizona, dehumidifiers are not installed.
4. Control effectiveness testing, measurement, or observation
   The effectiveness of the control is measured with electronic sensors.
5. Testing frequency or sampling plans
   Measurements are made at the beginning and end of each shift.
6. The functional area that is responsible for the control processes or procedures
   Humidity control systems are operated by Facility Engineering.
7. The functional area that is responsible for observing, measuring, or testing the effectiveness of control
   Humidity is monitored by Facility Engineering.
8. The range of acceptable process control limits: specifications; normal, alert, and action levels
   specification = 20–65% RH
   October–May normal = 30–40% RH
   alert = 25–30% RH; 40–50% RH
   action = 20–25% RH; 50–60% RH
   June–September normal = 40–50% RH
   alert = 30–40% RH; 50–55% RH
   action = 20–30% RH; 55–60% RH
9. Any predetermined response to common deviations
   When the humidity is lower than 20%, as there is no humidification in the system, clean the area to increase the moisture content.
10. Identification of critical/essential control points, validated limits, or acceptance criteria that will assist in the triage of data-of-exception observations
    Humidity control in manufacturing areas is not considered a CCP or ECP for current production operations.

Note: Although humidity control is useful as an example, it is usually one of several environmental quality characteristics that are controlled, and information monitoring programs are written to encompass all environmental control monitoring requirements, e.g., bioburden, nonviable particles, temperature, air pressure differentials, etc.

Establish information monitoring programs in controlled documents. Monitoring program documents with pre-determined formats assure consistency of program content, monitoring criteria, monitoring limits, and trending requirements. An example is provided in Exhibit 3.2.

NORMAL OPERATING CONDITIONS, ALERT LIMITS, ACTION LIMITS, AND SPECIFICATIONS

A clear understanding of normal operating conditions is essential to the establishment of good control limits. Process control limits should be:
- linked to associated product/process disposition, meaning that when values are within limits the product/process is acceptable, and when values are not within limits the product/process is unacceptable
- associated with products/processes that are/can be controlled, meaning that monitoring values are likely to fall within acceptable limits.

Although the primary purpose of process control limits is to indicate when a product or process is unacceptable, they can also be used to prevent failure when they are expanded to include alert and action limits. Alert and action limits are control points between normal and unacceptable that represent warning limits for potential problems. Warning limits provide time to investigate and resolve problems before they have any real impact on product or processing.

Establish information monitoring program limits as follows:

Normal Operating Conditions are a range of values associated with the routine operating attributes, characteristics, or parameters. Normal operating condition values are obtained from experience with equipment, process, product, or environmental performance in the current configuration in the current environment of use.

Alert limits are a range of values that, when exceeded, signal a potential drift from normal operating conditions. Alert limit ranges fall between normal operating ranges and action limit ranges. When an alert limit is exceeded, more frequent monitoring may be required.

Action limits are a range of values that fall between alert limits and specifications that when exceeded signal an apparent drift from normal operating conditions. When the action limit range is reached, action is required. These actions should be predetermined.

Specifications are a range of values associated with operational attributes, characteristics, or parameters beyond which the process, product, equipment system, support utility (water, steam, air, gas), or environment, etc., is considered unacceptable for use.

INFORMATION MONITORING PROGRAM IMPLEMENTATION, TRAINING, AND DATA ENTRY MANAGEMENT

All information monitoring programs must be written by or in collaboration with the functional area that will perform routine monitoring. Information collected as directed in these monitoring programs must be used. Monitoring data confirms process control, supports troubleshooting efforts, and gathers information for future change.

The line worker or technician is the first line of defense in the management of risk. As a result, they must understand the difference between data-of-exception and data-of-compliance observations for each monitoring event. The records that support data collection in monitoring programs must be simple to use. When programs request redundant or excessive information collection, workers will take shortcuts and the effectiveness of the program will suffer.

Information monitoring programs should be managed day today by the functional areas in which the monitoring information is collected. These areas are responsible for fulfilling the scheduled commitments of the program and notifying the Formal Investigation Team and/or QA when Level II/III observations are made. Data-of-compliance observation trending from all programs is managed by Quality Assurance or some group that reports to Quality Assurance. Monitoring for adverse trends in data-of-compliance and data-of exception observations is an extension of the trending/auditing function.

Data-of-Compliance Trending

Information monitoring programs must manage both data-of-exception and data-of-compliance observations. Data-of-exception observations as discussed in this chapter are managed on an event-by-event basis and judged for their potential impact on product or process quality. Data-of-compliance observations are managed on a periodic basis and judged for their potential impact on product or process quality.

Trending data-of-compliance observations is a systematic process that specifies the data sets to be evaluated, the frequency of evaluation, the evaluation methods or statistical techniques used, and definitions for adverse trends in the data sets. When observations are generated from trend analysis, record these observations as data-of-exception and proceed as discussed in this chapter, i.e., confirm the observation, perform deviation triage, and conduct a Preliminary Investigation. Finally, when trends in the data are observed, share these observations with the workers in the area that collected the original information. This feedback will promote increased awareness in workers and is likely to provide insight into the cause of the trends (see Chapter 9).

Exhibit 3.1

Page __1__ of __2__

Out-of-Specification Result Observation and Preliminary Investigation Record

Observation ID# _____

Observation Record (Section A)

Date of Observation _____ Date of Event _____

ID# of Sample _____ Lot # _____

ID# of Test Method _____ Revision # _____

What SHOULD have been observed? _____

_____

_____

What was observed? _____

_____

_____

Does this observation   ( ) invalidate the test performed?   ( ) deviate from an ECP limit?
                                  ( ) trigger an alert limit?   ( ) deviate from a PCP limit?
                                  ( ) trigger an action limit?
                                  ( ) deviate from an established specification?
                                  ( ) deviate from a finished product specification?

Where is the limit/specification that "should have been met" documented?

                 Document ID# _____ Version _____

Proposed cause for the observation _____

Note: "When clear evidence of lab error exists . . . testing results should be invalidated." (FDA/OOSR Guide)

( ) Submit this form to Supervisor or Manager in your functional area.

Observer _____ Department _____ Date _____ Time _____

Observation Confirmation (Section B)

Confirm observation as   ( ) invalid test; provide retest instructions below;
                                      cross out remainder of form
                            ( ) alert/action limit violation; conduct preliminary investigation
                            ( ) out-of-specification result; conduct preliminary investigation

Is there enough of the original sample remaining to conduct a retest? ( ) yes   ( ) no

Instructions/Comments _____

Verified by _____ Date _____ Time _____

Exhibit 3.1 (continued)

Out-of-Specification Result Observation and Preliminary Investigation Record

Page __2__ of __2__

Preliminary Investigation (Section C)

What was investigated/evaluated? Consider the potential for:
- ( ) Equipment calibrations or performance failure
- ( ) Reagent performance failure
- ( ) Sample handling deviations or sample deterioration
- ( ) Technician training deficiencies
- ( ) Product Risk Analysis and CCP/ECP designations
- ( ) Method deviations
- ( ) Calculation errors

Observations from Preliminary Investigation: _____
_____
_____

Has cause been determined? ( ) yes ( ) no   If so, indicate cause here _____
_____

Observation Triage (Section D)

Assign a level-of-concern to this observation.

( ) Level III — Observations require immediate Formal Investigation and notification of QA and Regulatory. Level III OOSR events include stability study test failures for commercial product stored at recommended storage conditions, or any event which compromises the safety of product already in the market.

( ) Level II — Observations require Formal Investigation because cause is not known and must be known to take effective action.

( ) Level I — Observations have a predefined response indicated in procedures (alert and action limits), or observation cause is known and easily corrected.

   ( ) Direct Action Implementation _____
   _____

   ( ) Alert/Action Limit actions as proposed in Document ID# _____ version ___

Supervisor/Manager _____ Date _____ Time _____

Notification

Level II/III: deliver to QA   Date _____ Time _____ Rec'd by _____

Level I: copy to Action Database

Supervisor/Manager _____ Date _____ Time _____

Exhibit 3.2

Page __1__ of __3__

Environmental Monitoring Program Document Example

1.0 Purpose and Scope – Describe the objective of the monitoring program and what it applies to or does not apply to within the facility or department.

This program identifies the environmental monitoring requirements for temperature, humidity, air flow, air pressure, particulates, and bioburden in Clean Room 88.

2.0 Responsibility/Training – Declare who is responsible for fulfilling the directives of this program and who is responsible for data assessment and reporting requirements.

Quality Assurance is responsible for the design of this monitoring program; individual responsibilities for monitoring are detailed in 4.0 and 6.0.

3.0 Control Parameters, Specifications, and Methods – Control parameters are measures and conditions associated with processes, equipment, utilities, environments, etc., that have the potential to adversely affect product. List the control parameters that can be observed or measured routinely to assess the effectiveness of this control.

3.1 Control Parameters

Parameters: temperature, relative humidity, air flow, air pressure between adjacent rooms, bioburden, particulates.

3.2 Control Mechanisms

3.2.1 Temperature, humidity, air flow, and air pressure *are maintained by a constant volume HVAC system with a terminal reheat, a chemical dehumidifier, and a steam grid humidifier. Conditioned air is filtered through a series of prefilters and final HEPA filters designed to remove 99.997% of particles of 0.3 microns. Rooms are balanced to achieve air pressurization and air flow requirements.*

3.2.2 Bioburden *is controlled by the supply of clean air to the area, the maintenance of humidity levels, and a rigorous cleaning and disinfection program (SOP 451).*

3.2.3 Particulate levels *are maintained with HEPA filters supplying clean air to the area and with a cleaning and disinfection program.*
The facility maintenance engineer is responsible for the operation and maintenance of this equipment and for the cleaning and disinfection programs.

4.0 Monitoring Methods and Sampling Schedules – What are the methods for monitoring the effectiveness of maintenance? For each parameter listed, reference a procedure which details the test methods, sample handling requirements, and sampling plans (sample size, frequency, sample sites).

4.1 *Temperature, humidity, air flow, and air pressure are measured electronically with the Climet® Control System. These values are recorded continuously onto an electronic medium and are read manually once a day and recorded in the Clean Room Environmental Logbook located in the control room. Monitoring of these parameters is the responsibility of the Quality Engineer.*

Exhibit 3.2 (continued)

Page __2__ of __3__

Environmental Monitoring Program Document Example

4.2 Bioburden levels in air are measured with a slit sampler according to SOP 3211. Daily monitoring occurs before work begins in the area and weekly when there is no work scheduled for the area. Sampling is performed at the work bench and at least 10 ft^3 of air is sampled. Bioburden sampling and testing are the responsibility of the Microbiologist.

4.3 Particulate levels are measured with a Met One portable sampler according to SOP 4566. Daily monitoring occurs before work begins in the area and weekly when there is no work scheduled for the area. Sampling is performed at the work bench and in the gowning area; at least 20 ft^3 of air is sampled. Particulate sampling and testing is the responsibility of the Quality Engineer.

5.0 Standards – If the corporate standards listed in this document are based on any harmonized standards or compendial standards, list those sources; e.g., Environmental control standards are based on USP 24 recommendations and monitoring experience in Clean Room 88 since 6/98.

Parameter	Specification	Normal
Temperature	62–77F	68–70C
Relative Humidity	20–55%	30–40%
Air Flow	laminar	laminar
	90 ft/min +/- 20% across filter	90–110 ft/min
	550–650 air changes/hour	570–600
Air Pressure diff. adjacent rooms	positive flow to outside;	0.02–0.05" water
Bioburden	< 10 CFU/10 ft^3	1–2CFU/10 ft^3
Particulates	< 100 particles/ft^3 > 0.5µ	0–20 particle/ft^3

Parameter	Alert Limits	Action Limits
Temperature	65–67F; 71–73F	62–64F; 74–76F
Relative Humidity	20–30%; 40–45%	45–55%
Air Flow	NA	nonlaminar
	NA	72–89; 101–107 ft/min
	NA	550–569; 601–649 air changes/hour
Air Pressure diff. adjacent rooms	0.010–0.019" water 0.050–0.060" water	< 0.010" water > 0.060" water
Bioburden	3–5 CFU/ft^3	6–9 CFU/ft^3
Particulates	21–50 particles/ft^3 > 0.5µ	51–99 particles/ft^3 > 0.5µ

6.0 Data Collection and Data Management – Describe data collection methods and data handling requirements. Consult information about alert and action levels, below.

> Daily particulates and bioburden values are calculated in ft^3, and these values are recorded in the Clean Room Logbook. The Quality Engineer is responsible for data collection.

> Temperature, humidity, air flow, and air pressure values are reviewed daily. If temperature and humidity values are within required limits for 20 out of 24 hours, they are considered acceptable. If air pressures maintain a positive flow and all adjacent rooms have at least a 0.05" differential, they are considered acceptable. If air changes/hour fall within requirements with no excursions of more than 700 or less than 400, it is considered acceptable. The Quality Engineer is responsible for data collection.

Exhibit 3.2 (continued)

Page __3__ of __3__

Environmental Monitoring Program Document Example

7.0 Data Review and Reporting Requirements – Indicate any requirements to notify management and the actions that must be taken when monitoring data do not meet requirements. Indicate who is responsible for reporting.

- When data is within an alert/action level, record the observation as a Level I observation according to SOP 4711 and take actions described in specific, monitoring SOP.
- When data is out-of-specification, record the observations as Level II observations according to SOP 4711.
- No Level III observations are expected from this monitoring program.

8.0 Deviation Management Information
Critical Control Points (CCPs) for the Environmental Monitoring Program, depending on the product processed in the Clean Room, include:

- Air pressure differential loss or reversed direction of flow (<=0" water) in filling suite during aseptic filling.
- Bioburden limits exceeded in the filling suite, at level of filling operation or above, during aseptic filling operations.

CHAPTER 4

RISK-BASED DECISION MAKING FOR POST-MARKET FEEDBACK INFORMATION MONITORING PROGRAMS

Monitoring for information associated with product use in the patient or user environments does not end when clinical studies are completed and market authorization is granted. Regulatory authorities and consumers expect that products in the market will be monitored to identify unexpected Adverse Events and that the surveillance programs will be designed to alert authorities and users to potential threats to public health.

Post-market feedback programs monitor the market through complaint programs, post-market clinical studies, observations collected during customer support activities, articles published by product users, etc. Information collected by these activities and programs ranges from formal complaints to the casual comments made by product users to company representatives. No matter what the source or format of the information and no matter how the information is transmitted to the company, there should be a consistent approach to the collection and management of this information.

"The specific objectives of FDA's postmarketing risk assessment programs are to detect Adverse Events not previously observed, improve understanding of the potential severity of previously anticipated risks, detect events resulting from . . . effects in particular populations and assess the potential for causal relationships."(1)

Design information monitoring programs to collect and assess product performance and product usage, throughout a product's life, in its environment of use. Use this information to identify:
- Adverse Events
- unexpected product performance
- unexpected product usage practices.

As suggested in Chapter 3 and illustrated in Figure 3.1, information collected from the market should be processed systematically. Consider the following steps.

1) Determine whether the information is a data-of-exception observation, meaning that it represents an unexpected and/or unacceptable event, or if the information is a data-of-compliance observation, meaning that it represents an expected or acceptable event.

2) When the observation is determined to be a data-of-exception observation, a Preliminary Evaluation should be performed by a company representative, e.g., complaint handler, to:
- review the observation
- assign a level-of-concern to the observation based on predetermined risks associated with the observed problem and any associated decision trees in, for example, complaint handling procedures
- resolve those issues and problems that do not require Formal Investigation
- document the observation and the results of the Preliminary Evaluation
- notify QA when further investigation is warranted.

Monitoring Programs for Post-market Feedback Information

Complaint monitoring for Adverse Events

Medical product manufacturers/distributors are required to establish post-market monitoring programs that capture customer's complaints and identify Adverse Events about distributed products.

Complaints are any written, electronic, or oral communications that allege deficiencies related to the identity, quality, durability, reliability, safety, effectiveness, or performance of a product after it has been released for distribution.

Adverse Events are any unfavorable or unintended medical occurrence in a patient or subject associated with the use of a medical product, whether or not it is considered related to the medical product.

Complaints are evaluated on an event-by-event basis, as discussed below, to determine:

1) if they are data-of-exception or data-of-compliance observations
2) if data-of-exception observations are Adverse Events
3) if Adverse Events are Serious Adverse Events.

Serious Adverse Events are any adverse events associated with the use of the product resulting in:
- death
- life-threatening illness
- permanent disability
- inpatient hospitalization or continued hospitalization
- congenital anomaly
- required intervention to prevent permanent impairment.

Regulatory authorities expect that information monitoring programs designed to collect information from the market, such as complaint programs, alert the manufacturer/distributor, on an event-by-event basis, when:
- an unexpected Adverse Event occurs
- an anticipated Adverse Event or product failure occurs with increased frequency (when compared to the baseline frequency identified at the time of market approval)
- a marketed medical product is associated with a life-threatening or fatal event (a Serious Adverse Event).

Regulatory authorities expect a prompt and appropriate response that limits further exposure to products that have been associated with seriously unsafe conditions, and they expect to be notified of Serious Adverse Events. These expectations are established in regulations and guidelines (2-21).

Reporting systems for Adverse Event monitoring systems or programs in the U.S. include:
- AERS — Adverse Event Reporting System for drugs and therapeutic biologics
- CEARS — CBER Errors and Accidents Reporting System for the manufacture of biological products
- MDRs — Medical Device Reporting for device and diagnostic products
- DQRS — Drug Quality Reporting System for deviations from GMP that occur during manufacturing, shipping, or storage of prescription and over-the-counter drugs.
- Medication Error Reports — for errors that occur when prescribing, repacking, dispensing or administering a product
- MAUDE — Manufacturing and User Device Experience Database.

Other post-market feedback. There are additional routes of information flow that can be used to identify unexpected Adverse Events, and to further delineate already identified risks. They include:
- post-approval clinical studies
- post-market surveillance programs
- distributor and user reports
- physician experiences (verbal or published)
- company representative experiences with customers
- proceedings from scientific meetings
- other published literature.

This information should be collected and reviewed periodically. Data-of-exception observations should be culled from the information, recorded and evaluated as discussed below.

Preliminary Evaluation of Complaints

All complaints and market information are evaluated. This Preliminary Evaluation is conducted by a company representative, e.g., complaint handler, as soon as possible after the event has been observed. During the Preliminary Evaluation, the observation is reviewed, information about the observation is gathered to determine an appropriate level-of-concern, and the observation is either managed according to predetermined procedures, or it is referred to the Formal Investigation Team (Chapter 5).

Complaint Review and Information Gathering

All complaints must be reviewed by a company representative. The questioning that supports this review process should provide the first opportunity to characterize the concern or problem, identify its cause, and take appropriate action when authorized, e.g., Direct Action Implementation (Chapter 6). Consider the following review elements:
- Confirm whether the product is involved in the observation and, if possible, identify the product specifically (lot number).
- Interview the individual who observed the issue, deviation, or problem about what they observed.
- Review any documentation of the event generated by the patient or the user. Is there evidence of product failure?
- Review equipment performance records, reagent identification and performance records, and personnel training records to ensure their adequacy.
- Look for product usage deviations. Ensure that the correct procedure was used and the most recent version of the method. Interview the

observer about the procedure to ensure that it was followed. Indicate if this is the first use of a new procedure or a new version.
- Observe samples or returned product, when appropriate. Is it completely and correctly identified? Indicate when there is anything about the product or the sample that would suggest that it was improperly handled.
- Assign a level-of-concern to the observation, as directed in company procedures and/or decision trees (see below).

Questioning techniques for complaint handlers. As discussed in Chapter 3, complete information gathering is essential to good investigational technique. As a result, the questioning associated with a Preliminary Evaluation of complaints and market information is expected to collect information about the observations without jumping to proposed causes or conclusions. This is facilitated in Operations by providing a predetermined set of questions in an information collection record (Exhibit 3.1) and training employees in the associated procedures. When collecting information about a problem from individuals outside of the company, however, the need for systematic questioning is even more critical to the success of the evaluation. Poorly worded questions can bias answers; vague questions can lead to conclusions instead of information about direct observations; inadequate questioning can lead to incomplete information. Design product-specific question forms for use by complaint handlers and train these individuals to interact effectively with observers outside the company. Specific, systematic questioning is essential in the collection of accurate, complete, and unbiased information.

COMPLAINT TRIAGE

Not all complaints represent data-of-exception observations; not all data-of-exception observations represent Adverse Events; not all Adverse Events are serious and reportable. Sorting complaints, market observations, and events is necessary to assure that the observations are relayed in a timely manner to the individuals most equipped to solve the problem. Complaint triage is designed to assign priority to the observations, based on the perceived impact that the observation might have on the safety or performance of the product, patient safety, or market stability. All complaints that represent data-of-exception observations are categorized into levels-of-concern based on organization-wide, risk analysis for products (Chapter 1) and based on regulations.

As suggested in Chapter 3, three levels-of-concern are proposed for triage:

Level III — Level III observations include any Serious Adverse Events that are reportable. They require *immediate* investigation and action.

Level II — Level II observations include any product failures or Adverse Events. Level II observations might require Formal Investigation to determine cause, and take corrective or preventive action, but many Level II observations have predefined responses provided in decision trees based on regulatory requirements. Level II Adverse Events may be reportable if they represent an increased frequency or increased severity of a problem.

Level I — These data-of-exception observations have no impact on patient safety or product performance, or there are predefined responses to these deviations provided in decision trees and procedures. Level I assignments are appropriate when cause is known and corrective action is obvious and easily implemented. Data-of-exception observation records should be designed to facilitate the close-out of all Level I observations by providing a record of the actions taken, and/or the rationale for not taking action at the completion of a Preliminary Evaluation.

The triage process for complaints and other market information should proceed as follows:

Distinguishing Data-of-Exception Observations from Data-of-Compliance Observations. The first decision required when collecting information about a marketed product is, "Can it be ignored for now and reviewed later, or must it be processed immediately?" Pre-established criteria in procedures and decision-trees to distinguish data-of-exception observations from data-of-compliance observations provide an observer with a quick and easy route of analysis. Compliance and exception for product performance and usage is based on product labeling, information-for-use instructions, package inserts, user manuals, and any other documents that accompany the product in the market and make claims about its use and performance. Data-of-compliance observations are collated to facilitate their use by Product Development, Customer Service, and Formal Investigation Teams. Data-of-exception observations are evaluated on an event-by-event basis.

Distinguishing Adverse Events from Data-of-Exception Observations. All the information collected about data-of-exception observations identified from complaints or other market information monitoring programs/studies is evaluated to identify Adverse Events. When Adverse Events are identified from complaints, the observation is moved to the next triage level (Level II); when an observation is not an Adverse Event, it is assigned to Level I.

Distinguishing Serious Adverse Events from Adverse Events. All Adverse Events are evaluated to identify Serious Adverse Events and determine the associated reporting requirements. When Serious Adverse Events and Reportable Events are identified from Adverse Events, they are assigned to Level III. All other Adverse Events remain assigned to Level II.

Serious Adverse Events associated with product use from any source are Reportable Events (2-20). Reportable Events are events that reasonably suggest that a product has or may have caused or contributed to a death, serious injury, or has malfunctioned and if the malfunction recurs it is likely to lead to serious injury or death. This includes any information that "might materially influence the benefit:risk assessments of a . . . product or that would be sufficient to consider changes in" product usage (20).

Decision Trees

Decision trees are established to facilitate routine decision making and to establish consensus expectations for observation triage. Decision trees are particularly useful in handling product complaints and identifying Adverse Events because there are detailed regulatory expectations for these decision-making processes. Decision trees can be used to distinguish data-of exception observations from data-of-compliance observations, Adverse Events from serious adverse events, Reportable Events from nonreportable events, and levels-of-concern (Levels I, II, III). See Exhibit 4.1.

Preliminary Evaluation Records and Notification

There should be a record of each Preliminary Evaluation, indicating that it was conducted as directed. The record should be accompanied by any additional information gathered from interviewing the observer to assist further investigation. Level I observation records, e.g., complaint records, should be submitted for entry into an action database as suggested in the Direct Action Implementation option in Chapter 6. Level II and Level III Preliminary Evaluation Records must be transferred to the Formal Investigation Team as soon as possible.

Action Implementation

As discussed in Chapter 6, there are two routes for action implementation. One route is quick and usually predetermined, allowing for immediate response to anticipated observations. This quick response route is beneficial in the management of complaints and Adverse Events because the reporting time frames can be as short as 5 days. A second route of action implementation involves a written protocol (Action Implementation Planning Protocols) that facilitates complex or critical action implementation requirements.

Actions Taken Before Investigations Are Complete

Reportable Events often require that action (in the form of reporting) be taken before an investigation to discover cause and propose effective actions has been completed. As suggested in Chapter 5, this may be necessary, but reporting an observation does not necessarily mean that the investigation is closed. Actions taken to comply with regulatory reporting requirements are not actions considered sufficient or complete to correct or prevent problems. Formal Investigations (Chapter 5) should be required for all Level III and Level II observations, as designated. Actions proposed from Formal Investigations are implemented and their effectiveness assessed as presented in Chapter 6.

Trending Data-of-Exception and Data-of-Compliance Observations

All complaints, Adverse Events, and Serious Adverse Events should be trended and analyzed for potential problems. To facilitate trend analysis, a library of product failure codes is developed, and a code is assigned to each failure. If a product risk analysis has been done, creating this library involves simply looking up the list of likely failure modes on the product risk analysis report.

Action taken in response to a report of increased frequency of an Adverse Event or product failure should depend on the severity of the Adverse Event or potential hazard associated with the product failure. It is tempting to minimize the severity under pressure of a possible product recall. As a result, decision making is more objective if the severity of the Adverse Event has already been established, e.g., in the Product Risk Analysis Report. Complaint handling procedures should direct the use of information from Product Risk Analysis Reports. An SOP might state, for example, "if the adverse effect is labeled 'Critical' on the product risk analysis table and the complaint trend report shows a 2x or greater increase in frequency, action to remove all product from the market that is within the scope of the problem must be taken immediately."

Actions Taken in the Market

Actions to reduce public exposure to unsafe products should be considered when an investigation reveals that:
- a marketed product has been associated with a life-threatening Adverse Event,
- an unexpected Adverse Event occurs, or
- an anticipated Adverse Event or product failure is occurring with increased frequency compared to the baseline frequency identified at the time of market approval.

Under these circumstances, the company must decide whether to continue to distribute the product, recall already distributed product, and/or halt further distribution until the problem is corrected. These are fundamental profit vs. safety decisions. The rationale for these decisions, and their implementation and effectiveness must be documented (Chapter 6).

RISK ANALYSIS UPDATES WITH POST-MARKET INFORMATION

Complaint handling procedures should require that reports of unexpected Adverse Events be added to the product risk analysis report and the severity of the adverse effect should be categorized following the product risk analysis procedure (see Chapter 1). To ensure objectivity, the risk analysis should be undertaken by a qualified group independent of those who must decide how to respond to the report.

CITED REFERENCES

1. U.S. Food and Drug Administration. "Managing Risks from Medical Product Use: Creating a Risk Management Framework," May 1999.
2. 21 CFR 310.305 — Records and reports concerning adverse drug experiences on marketed prescription drugs for human use without approved new drug applications.
3. 21 CFR 312.32 — Investigational new drug safety reports.
4. 21 CFR 314.80 — Postmarketing reporting of adverse drug experiences.
5. 21 CFR 314.81 — Other postmarketing reports (field alerts).
6. 21 CFR 806 — Corrections and removals.
7. 21 CFR 600.14 — Reporting of errors (biologics).
8. 21 CFR 600.80 — Postmarketing reporting of adverse experiences (for licensed biological products).
9. 21 CFR 803 — Medical device reporting.
10. 21 CFR 803.30 — Medical device reporting; Individual adverse event reports: User facilities.
11. 21 CFR 803.30 — Medical device reporting; Individual adverse event reports: Manufacturers.
12. 21 CFR 804 — Medical device distributor reporting.
13. 21 CFR 806 — Medical devices; reports of corrections and removals.
14. Reporting Serious Adverse Events and Product Problems with Human Drug and Biological Products and Devices (MEDWATCH); 58 FR 31596; June 3, 1993.
15. U.S. Food and Drug Administration. "Post-Marketing Reporting of Adverse Drug Experiences." March 1992.
16. U.S. Food and Drug Administration. "Post-marketing Reporting of Adverse Experiences—Biologics." October 1993.

17. U.S. Food and Drug Administration. "Post-Marketing Adverse Experience Reporting for Human Drug and Licensed Biological Products Clarification of What to Report." August 1997.
18. U.S. Food and Drug Administration. "Medical Device Reporting for Manufacturers." March 11, 1998.
19. U.S. Food and Drug Administration. "Medical Device Reporting for User Facilities." April 1, 1996.
20. U.S. Food and Drug Administration. "Medical Device Reporting: An Overview." April 1, 1996.
21. U.S. Food and Drug Administration. "Medical Device Reporting for Distributors." April 1, 1996.
22. "E2A Clinical Safety Data Management: Definitions and Standards for Expedited Reporting." March 1, 1995.
23. "E2C Clinical Safety Data Management: Periodic Safety Updates Reports." May 19, 1997.
24. "Guidance for Industry: Clinical Safety Data Management: Definitions and Standards for Expedited Reporting." ICH E2A. March 1995.
25. European Commission. "Guidelines on Medical Device Vigilance System." MED DEV 2.12/1. Brussels, Belgium.

Exhibit 4.1

Decision Record: Data-of-Exception Observations from Post-Market Feedback Information

Page __1__ of __2__

Note: Use this form to support level-of-concern assignments for market feedback observations that represent "data of exception" (i.e., information that represents an unexpected and/or unacceptable event). Consult SOP 1234.

1. Describe the observation below, or ( ) attach the complaint/observation form to this record.

2. Does the information represent an adverse event (i.e., an unfavorable or unintended medical occurrence in a patient or subject associated with the use of a medical product, whether or not related to the medical product)? ( ) yes   ( ) no

    Provide rationale in the following box.

3. Is the adverse event a serious adverse event (i.e., a medical occurrence that resulted in death or is life-threatening, requires/extends hospitalization, results in significant or persistent disability, or is a congenital birth defect)? ( ) yes   ( ) no

    Provide rationale below or ( ) attach rationale to this record.

Exhibit 4.1 (continued)

Decision Record: Data-of-Exception Observations from Post-Market Feedback Information

Page __2__ of __2__

4. Level-of-Concern assignment:

List the information reviewed to determine the seriousness of the event and assign the level-of-concern, or attach it to this record.

_____   _____

_____   _____

_____   _____

Assign a level-of-concern:

[ ] Level III   The observation involves product that is in the market, either commercially or under clinical investigation, and a *serious* Adverse Event that either has occurred or may reasonably occur if the cause of the event is not corrected.

File original and provide copy to Investigation Team and Regulatory Affairs promptly.

[ ] Level II   The observation involves product that is in the market, either commercially or under clinical investigation, and a non-Serious Adverse Event that either has occurred or may reasonably occur if the cause of the event is not corrected.

File original and provide copy to Investigation Team.

[ ] Level I   The observation involves product that is in the market and there is no adverse event associated with the observation.

File original and provide copy to QA.

_____   _____   _____

Signature of person making this decision   Title   Date

_____   _____   _____

Verification   Title   Date

CHAPTER 5

RISK-BASED DECISION MAKING IN FORMAL INVESTIGATION, ACTION IDENTIFICATION, AND AUTHORIZATION

Risk-based decision making is required to assure effective, efficient resolution of a company's most serious problems in a manner that complies with regulatory expectations for investigation and change control, assures product safety, and promotes profitability. Formal Investigations are conducted when the problem has not been resolved during Preliminary Investigations (Chapter 3) and/or when the data-of-exception observation could affect product safety and performance. In the language of this text, Formal Investigations are conducted for Level II and Level III data-of-exception observations.

Every company that strives to comply with Good Manufacturing Practices, Quality System Regulations, or ISO 9000 Quality System Standards has procedures that direct the conduct of an investigation. These procedures establish when investigations are required, who is responsible, and what documentation is required to provide evidence that the procedures were followed. Seldom, however, does an investigation procedure describe how to investigate a problem. It is a common assumption that if enough smart people are assembled in a room to solve a problem they will discover cause. This assumption ignores the fact that the basis of a good investigation is systematic processing of information and risk-based decision making about proposed actions by trained investigators.

This chapter presents phases of work associated with Formal Investigation (also called Failure Investigation in some regulations) and presents action identification practices. The next chapter will present the work associated with action implementation practices.

FORMAL INVESTIGATION CRITERIA

Data-of-exception observations provide evidence that something is not as it is expected to be, i.e., out-of-specification results, unexpected observations, procedural deviations, discrepancies, or nonconforming units. All data-of-exception observations are investigated as discussed in Chapter 3 under Preliminary Investigation. Some data-of-exception observations require further analysis, called Formal Investigation, to determine the cause and to identify corrective/preventive actions. Formal Investigations are conducted for data-of-exception observations:
- not resolved during Preliminary Investigations
- likely to affect the safety, performance or quality of products, manufacturing processes, or test methods
- for which cause is not known
- that require the determination of cause to take effective action.

Example: While driving down the road your car suddenly loses power and stops running. As you pull to the side of the road you look at the control panel and notice, with amazement, that the gas gauge indicates "empty." Do you need to investigate? No; the cause is known.

Example: Walking into the house one day you discover that the power is off in the kitchen. You quickly walk to the breaker panel and notice that the breaker #3 has been tripped. You turn it on and the power is restored. Do you need to investigate? No; you do not need to know cause to take corrective action. You may, as will be discussed later, investigate to take preventive action if you are worried about the problem recurring.

FORMAL INVESTIGATION TEAMS

The Formal Investigation Team is a group of individuals who perform their analysis and decision making from the technical perspective of the product/process design. Team members represent the major disciplines of the environment in which the problems occur. When observations from the commercial manufacturing operation are investigated, the team would include Technical Services/Validation, Quality Control, Quality Assurance, Materials Management, Maintenance, and various Manufacturing groups. When observations from the market (complaints or Adverse Events) are investigated, the team would include Marketing, Customer Service, Clinical Affairs, Quality Assurance, Product Development, and Regulatory.

Team members should be at the supervisory or manager level (depending on the size of the company), but they should not be chosen based on position alone. Investigations take time and dedication; ensure that investigators are good technically, have an inquisitive nature, and are willing to invest time in the team. Ensure that those who manage investigation team members, normally, understand the cost and the value of their services to the company. Management must be willing to support the time away from routine work required by team members to do good investigations.

Define a minimum membership for the group, and alternate members. Train this group, as a group, in the investigation process. As will be discussed in subsequent chapters, the success of the team is directly affected by its ability to perform quickly, under pressure, and with confidence. Positive group dynamics are essential to this mission and consistent, rigorous training and development is required. (For further information see Chapter 8: Managing Groups that Manage Risk.)

Team leadership should be established and remain consistent for extended periods of time. In large organizations consider Quality Assurance for this leadership position; and when possible, retain their leadership as a nonvoting member of the group. If this cannot be done, identify a third party within the organization or a consultant (who can be used when needed) to facilitate discussions of complex or difficult problems. The third-party individual must also be trained with the group.

FORMAL INVESTIGATION TEAM MEETINGS

Every meeting should follow a fixed agenda. Common agenda items from meeting to meeting include review of new problems and review of previously analyzed problems at various phases of investigation.

There are many rules of conduct and meeting format considerations that can have an impact on the performance and efficiency of the team. Although these will be discussed in greater detail in Chapter 8, consider the following:

- In every phase of investigation, solicit input from each member of the investigation team. Establish a meeting agenda that makes this a routine expectation.
- Information presented in meetings should be presented in written form (provided to members days before the meeting begins) and presented in visual form as it is discussed with the group. Consider rules that clarify the difference between information "I know" because there is data to support it and information "I think I know" because it is based on probabilities or conjecture.

- All information presented in a meeting should be provided to members before the meetings begin. All members must review these packages before the meetings. Individual assessments of information packages provide an invaluable perspective on problems and solutions that will be lost if information is only considered in group sessions.

The Formal Investigation Process

Every Level III observation and some Level II data-of-exception observations should move through all phases of investigation and action planning, even when cause is not determined and no action is recommended. Consider the following phases of investigation, analysis, and action (Exhibits 5.1, 5.2, 5.3):

Phase 1 – Investigation Initiation
Phase 2 – Gather Information for Problem Characterization
Phase 3 – Determine and Verify Cause
Phase 4 – Action Analysis and Action Authorization
Phase 5 – Action Implementation and Follow-up

Phase 1 – Investigation initiation and problem definition

In the first phase of investigation define the problem specifically, confirm its level-of-concern, and begin to characterize the problem according to the established procedures (Exhibit 5.1).

Define the problem. Data-of-exception observations must be clearly and completely defined in order to focus the information-gathering phase of the investigation. Make a simple statement that identifies the item that is having the problem and specifically describes the kind of trouble that has been observed.

Example: "The autoclave doesn't work." This statement identifies the object of investigation but it does not identify what is wrong. Be specific. Does the autoclave fail to start, does it fail to heat up to the specified temperature, does it fail to run the cycle as programmed, does it fail to shut off and allow the door to be open, does it fail to sterilize? What exactly is wrong with the autoclave? Also, if there is more than one autoclave in the facility, which autoclave?

Regulatory review. Initiate a regulatory review for all Level III observations and for Level II observations as needed. The regulatory review identifies any known, regulatory requirements associated with the data-of-exception observation, adverse events, and proposed actions. Initiating a regulatory review before the investigation is completed promotes risk-based decision making in the triage of observations and assures that regulatory obligations are met (Exhibit 5.4).

Triage confirmation and prioritization of investigations. Review information provided on the Data-of-Exception Observation Forms and/or the Preliminary Investigation records from Operations or the Complaint Handling form from Customer Service. Confirm or change the level assignment of the observation by reviewing any guidance provided in product risk analysis reports or CCP/ECP identifications for processes in batch records, monitoring program documents, etc. If a level assignment is changed, provide a rationale.

Level assignment for observations also serves to prioritize the work of the Formal Investigation Team, as Level III observations should always take precedence over other, ongoing investigations.

Phase 2 – Gathering of Information for Problem Characterization

Information gathering is the most important phase of the investigative process. When the information is accurate and complete, cause is often apparent at the conclusion of this phase. The information-gathering phase *must be complete*. If one jumps to conclusions or proposes a cause before all information is collected, it will be difficult to verify a most probable cause when the investigation is concluded. If one proposes cause before information is collected to characterize the problem, the information collection process is biased to support proposed cause.

The information-gathering phase is facilitated by establishing a list of questions to answer for every investigation. These questions are designed to define the observed problem as completely as possible. Gathering information to answer these questions may require additional testing, record review, and consultation with observers and/or functional area experts. Information-gathering questions and practices for observations in Operations differ from information-gathering questions and practices in Customer Service. Develop separate procedures and forms to facilitate these similar but different processes.

Information gathering should include, as standard practice, a search of data-of-exception entries from previous Formal Investigations for similar issues. This comparative information can be used to identify recurring problems or periodic problems.

Information gathering should be systematic. Ask questions about the object of the observation/problem and the unexpected characteristics of what was observed. Ask what, where, when, how much, how often? Answer all of these established questions; an example form is provided in Exhibit 5.1.

Information gathering should include a search for other similar products, equipment, processes, or users that could be having the same problems but are not (1). If discovered, determine the difference between what is observed to perform properly and the observed exception. Such differences often lead an investigator to discover the cause of a problem.

> ***Example:*** *Suppose you are watching TV and the screen turns fuzzy. What are you likely to do? You will probably switch channels. If only one channel has the problem, you are likely to conclude that the problem is with the channel and not with your TV set. If all channels are fuzzy, you are likely to conclude that the problem is with the TV set. To verify this you might try another TV set in the house.*

Information gathering should identify things that have changed at about the same time the problem was first noticed. This allows a comparison of before-and-after that can focus the investigation on what has changed. Similarly, information gathering should identify the difference between products, equipment, users, and processes that perform successfully and those that do not; this also can focus the investigation on probable cause. (1)

> ***Example:*** *While walking into the house one cold winter evening, you reach to turn on the porch light and nothing happens. You walk cautiously through the house and try to turn on the table lamp; again, no light comes on. You walk to the bedroom, flip on another switch, and the bedroom light goes on!*
>
> *Quickly you analyze the problem. You have already gathered information about the problem. The porch light and the table lamp have the problem but not the bedroom light.*
>
> *Next you ask what is different about the lights with the problem compared to the lights that do not have the problem. The answer is that the table lamp and the porch light are on the same circuit and the bedroom light is not.*
>
> *Finally you ask what has changed about the problem circuit compared to the trouble-free circuit. You remember that you plugged an electric space heater into that circuit this morning . . . probable cause identified!*

Record information gathered about a problem in a consistent format, e.g., an information gathering form (Exhibit 5.1). Consistency in data records will facilitate review of information by the investigators for the current investigation and future investigations.

Phase 3 – Determine and verify cause

Identify possible causes. Possible causes are those things or conditions that could lead to the characteristics of the problem as described in the problem definition/characterization form. Solicit possible causes from individual members of the Formal Investigative Team in writing *before* group discussion of probable cause occurs.

Initiate group discussion about possible causes with a list of possible causes submitted from the individual members of the group. Ensure that every member offers at least one possible cause *before* discussions begin. Identify *anything* that could possibly cause the observed event or data. Without several possible causes to consider, the decision-making process of the group can be biased.

Identify the most probable cause and verify. The most probable cause of a problem is identified by verifying that it makes sense in light of the information collected about the problem in Phase 2. For each proposed cause ask, "If this were the cause, would it explain the information gathered about what the problem affected, when the problem happened, where the problem occurred, and so on?"

From the list of possible causes that survive this checking event, identify the most probable cause. When possible design experiments or gather additional information to verify the most probable cause.

When cause is still not known. When an investigation is complete and cause is not determined or verified, do not invent a cause just to close the investigation. Although cause must be known to design corrective actions, not all investigations discover cause. There are, however, other actions that may be appropriate (adaptive actions) when cause is not known.

> *Example: It is discovered that a lyophilizer is leaking oil during a cycle. It is not possible to discover the cause of the leak until the cycle is completed, but if one keeps pouring oil into the compressor during the cycle the product will not be compromised. This is an adaptive action.*

When cause has not been discovered during investigation, develop a mechanism to mark the investigation as "cause not determined" for future reference. "Cause not determined" may occur when a deviation is a first event in a set of periodic problems, and a second deviation needs to occur before a time sequence can be used to discover cause. "Cause not determined" may also occur when the team must take action before cause is determined; it is sometimes necessary to make product or component disposition decisions and to take action before the investigation is closed. Similarly, reporting Adverse Events to regulatory authorities is an action that must be taken, often before the investigation is complete (Chapter 4).

Action Proposals. The Formal Investigation Team proposes actions based on its knowledge of the problem and its most probable cause. There may be more than one action required to solve a problem, and there may be more than one alternative for every action. All proposed actions and their associated alternatives should be listed for review.

When actions are proposed, it is useful if the Formal Investigation Team also considers any adverse consequences associated with alternative actions because this information will facilitate a more knowledgeable action analysis review.

Action is not always required or recommended. If no action is required this recommendation and its rationale must be documented.

Phase 4 – Action analysis and action authorization

Action analysis. All actions proposed in association with Level III observations and some proposed actions associated with Level II observations (upon request of the Formal Investigation Team) are reviewed by the Action Analysis Team before action implementation can proceed. Action analysis is suggested when proposed actions involve the expenditure of significant money, time, or resources, or when actions might affect the patient, product user, or market. Such analysis must also consider the information provided by the Regulatory Review Record, initiated during Phase 1.

The Action Analysis Team decides between several proposed actions when more than one option is available. If and when an action is confirmed as appropriate, the action is "identified." The Action Analysis Team must identify actions *and* authorize their implementation before action implementation can proceed. Actions can be grouped for implementation under an Action Implementation Planning Protocol or implemented as single events (Direct Action Implementation), discussed in Chapter 6.

- **Why Two Teams? Formal Investigation Team vs. and Action Analysis Team**
Actions proposed by the Formal Investigation Team, from a technical, operational, or patient/user perspective, do not consider the impact that such actions might have on the business. The Action Analysis Team is responsible for considering the action proposals of the Formal Investigation Team with the added perspective of business values and priorities.

As a result Action Analysis Team members are different from investigators; they must be or represent management in the areas of operation where the problems occur and where impact of the problem is likely to be observed. Functional area representation should include Quality Control, Manufacturing, Quality Assurance, Regulatory, Validation, Maintenance, Materials Management, Marketing, Customer Service, and Clinical Affairs.

- **Action Analysis Team Meetings**

Action Analysis Team meetings are scheduled to support Level III investigations because regulatory notification requirements can be as short as 5–15 days. If possible, Action Analysis Team members can sit in with the Formal Investigation Team when proposed actions are presented but *not* during the Formal Investigation process. Cooperative meetings of investigators and management can expedite information/knowledge transfer.

Action authorization. When proposed actions have been reviewed by the Action Analysis Team, the team authorizes the implementation of selected actions. Some proposed actions will not be selected; some proposed actions will be implemented at a later date, etc. The disposition of all proposed actions should be documented as suggested in Exhibit 5.3. It is also recommended that each authorized action be identified with a unique action identification number to facilitate tracking its history of implementation, monitoring, and effectiveness assessment.

Authorized actions are implemented through either Direct Action Implementation procedures or through Action Implementation Planning Protocols, discussed in Chapter 6. The priority of action implementation is declared when the action is authorized based on the seriousness, urgency, or priority of the associated problem, although some priorities are predetermined by regulatory authorities because of inherent safety or performance issues associated with the product. Factors that affect priority assignment can be derived from the Regulatory Review Record, product risk analysis reports, complaint handling records, and CCP/ECP assignments.

Providing a priority scale of high, medium, and low can facilitate the triage of actions that move through these team meetings. High priority can be defined, specifically, in company procedures; e.g., high priority actions should be implemented ASAP or within 5 days of action proposals. Consider the following actions as *high* priority:

- actions derived from Level III Observations, e.g., actions associated with Serious Adverse Events
- actions that require implementation before further production and testing can be conducted
- actions that require implementation before product can be released
- actions required to support regulatory commitments and 483 citation or warning letter responses.

Phase 5 – Action implementation and follow-up

Action Implementation. Identified authorized actions are implemented, as suggested by their priority assignment, in a systematic manner. Action implementation and effectiveness assessments are discussed in Chapter 6.

Always Ask: "What else?" When cause is discovered and corrective actions considered, the team must also consider what else might be affected by this cause and what else might go wrong because of this implemented action. The inquiry into what else could be affected by this cause extends the problem-solving efforts into the area of potential problem analysis because it considers whether the cause of one problem could be the potential cause of other similar problems. The inquiry into what else might go wrong because of this implemented action extends the problem-solving efforts into the area of risk analysis associated with any change, because changes to products and processes that are not evaluated for risk could create new problems while solving others.

Documentation, Logs, and Databases. Each "Formal Investigation Package" must contain the following:
- a copy of the original observation, complaint, deviation, etc. and associated Preliminary Investigation information
- the investigation record, +/– regulatory review record, +/– action analysis record
- extra testing conducted to gather information or verify cause
- proposed, identified, authorized actions.

Each investigation package should be filed in QA according to its ID number. In addition, an investigation log is required to manage the work of the Formal Investigation Team. This log should indicate the identity, category, and status of every investigation as it moves through the investigation process.

Formal investigation meeting minutes should be kept chronologically. The event-specific investigation record can simply cite the meeting dates when a specific problem was discussed and who participated in the meetings.

The Investigation Is Closed. Define the criteria that must be met before an investigation is considered closed. There are always regulatory expectations for the timeliness of investigations. Identify data-of-exception observation dates, investigation initiation dates, and investigation closure dates. Establish process controls or adopt recommended regulatory controls for the timeliness of investigations.

Defining when an investigation is closed is not easy. There are pitfalls for many of the possibilities. If, for example, an investigation is considered closed:
- before actions are taken:
  – then action implementation and effectiveness determinations can be neglected.
- after all actions associated with the investigation have been implemented:
  – then investigations can remain open for long periods of time, and determining the effectiveness of actions can be neglected.
- after the effectiveness of all associated with the investigation have been determined:
  – then investigations can remain open for months and years.

Given these issues, the closure of an investigation should be defined as the point at which actions have been authorized and a separate program should be developed to identify and track the implementation and follow-up of individual actions. This will be discussed in the next chapter.

The efficiency of the risk-based decision-making processes of observation triage, deviation investigation, and action implementation impacts the effectiveness of risk management. Develop useful, informative measures and controls for these processes that assure a timely response to problems and action taking.

CITED REFERENCE
1. Kepner-Tregoe. 1978. *Analytical Troubleshooting.* Princeton, NJ: Princeton University Press.

Exhibit 5.1

```
                                              Page  1  of  1
```

Information Gathering for Investigations in Operations

Investigation ID# _____

Level-of-Concern _____

What is having a problem? _____

What is wrong with it? _____

Information Gathering About the Problem

WHAT

_____   _____
_____   _____

WHERE

_____   _____
_____   _____

WHEN

_____   _____
_____   _____

HOW MUCH of it is affected

_____   _____
_____   _____

Are there comparisons to be made between what is affected by the problem and what is not affected, when it occurred and when it didn't occur, etc.?

If so, what are the differences between these items, times, etc.?

Are there any changes that could be related to the problem?

Are there previous problems, "cause not determined" investigations, etc., that could be related to this problem?

Attachments _____

Completed by _____   Date _____

Exhibit 5.2

Page __1__ of __3__

Formal Investigation Record

Section A — Investigation ID   Investigation ID# _____

Date investigation request was received _____   Observation ID# _____

Request origin = ( ) OOS event observation record;   Date of event = _____
( ) Deviation or audit observation;   Date of event = _____
( ) Complaint or adverse event;   Date of event = _____
( ) Other : _____ ;   Date of event = _____

Preliminary Level-of-Concern Assignments from Observer = Level _____

If a product disposition decision is likely to be affected by this investigation, confirm that the product is properly segregated and identified.

Product ID _____ Lot # _____ ( ) proper identification confirmed

QA _____ Date _____

Section B — Triage Confirmation

( ) 1. This investigation could lead to a decision to recall product from the market.
( ) 2. This investigation has been initiated because a patient or user has been seriously injured or could be seriously injured.
( ) 3. This investigation is likely to affect a product disposition decision.
Note: If #1 or #2 is checked, Level III must be assigned; if #3 is checked, Level II or III must be assigned.
( ) The Observation and/or Preliminary Investigation Record has been reviewed and the level-of-concern is determined to be _____.

Justification for any change to level-of-concern assignments from preliminary assignment:

_____
_____

QA/Investigation Team Member _____ Date _____

Section C — Regulatory Review

( ) For all Level III observations and Level II, as needed.
( ) not needed

QA/Investigation Team Member _____ Date Submitted_____

Exhibit 5.2 (continued)

Page __2__ of __3__

Formal Investigation Record

Section D — Investigation

First Failure Investigation Meeting held on _____ (date)

    ( ) Information Gathering for Investigation Record attached

    Subsequent Meeting dates _____
    _____
    _____

What is the Most Probable Cause? _____

What else could be affected by this cause?

    ( ) no other potential problems identified

    ( ) other potential problems include _____

Section E — Summary of Action Proposals, Action Identification, Action Authorization

( ) No action required; QA/Investigation Team Member _____ Date _____

Note: Action Summary log provided on page 3

QA/Investigation Team Member _____ Date _____

EXHIBIT 5.2 (CONTINUED)

Formal Investigation Record
Action Proposals, Action Identification, Action Authorization Summary

Page __3__ of __3__

*Action ID#	Proposed Action	Regulatory Review? (no/yes; date)	Action Analysis Team Review? (no/yes; date)	Proposed Actions that are identified (no/yes)	Action Implementation authorized (AIPP or Direct Action)

*Action ID#s are Investigation ID#s with a suffix of A, B, C, etc.

Product Development _____ Date _____ Quality Assurance _____ Date _____

Exhibit 5.3

Action Review Record

Investigation ID# _____ ; Level-of-concern assignment = Level _____

Page __1__ of __1__

Actions identified from this review:

Proposed Action ID#	Action Identified? (no/yes)	Priority for Implementation	Comments

Action Analysis Team Meetings

Date of meetings in which these actions were discussed _____

Actions suggested by Formal Investigation Team but *not* taken

Proposed Action _____ Rationale for no action _____
_____
_____

Completed by _____ Date _____

Exhibit 5.4

Page __1__ of __1__

Regulatory Review Record

Investigation ID# _____

Initial Regulatory Review Request Received on (date) _____

Problem Review Summary:

Does the problem trigger any regulatory concerns or notification/submission requirements to the regulatory authorities?

Proposed Actions Received for Review on (date) _____

Proposed Action Review Summary:

Do any of the proposed actions trigger any regulatory concerns or notification/submission requirements to the regulatory authorities?

Regulatory Review Performed by _____ Date _____

Verified by _____ Date _____

CHAPTER 6

RISK-BASED DECISION MAKING IN ACTION IMPLEMENTATION AND EFFECTIVENESS ASSESSMENT

Action implementation requires a rigorous and systematic approach. Without this discipline resources are wasted, problems that could be corrected continue, and changes are made in products and processes that have no positive impact. Action implementation has not been well managed, historically. FDA warning letters are filled with citations about actions that were never taken, action implementation tasks that were delayed for months, and actions taken that had no impact on the original problem. Action implementation and action effectiveness assessments have been ignored or poorly managed because the action implementation/effectiveness programs and the actions generated from the programs require additional and continuing organizational resources. Planning for the resources required to correct and prevent problems in operations or the market is seldom considered a necessary budget line item; if it is considered at all, it is underestimated because management plans for success, not failure.

When problems have been investigated and corrective actions identified (Chapter 5), management controls the resources needed to fix problems. If resources are scarce, budgets tight, or these concerns permeate the investigation process, information gathering and risk-based decision making will be biased toward the business priorities. When Formal Investigation and Action Implementation Procedures are designed with an independent management review element (as suggested in Chapter 5 with the Action Analysis Team), systematic bias of business priorities over technical problem solving is minimized. Then action implementation and action effectiveness assessments proceed efficiently and effortlessly, as presented in this chapter.

ACTION PLANNING

Not every investigation results in a proposed action; not every proposed action is implemented. When an investigation determines that no action is recommended, or when a proposed action is not confirmed upon review, this decision and the rationale for this decision must be documented. When actions have been identified and authorized for implementation, however, there should be two potential routes of implementation: one route of implementation should allow quick action with minimal documentation (Direct Action Implementation), and one route of implementation should provide for considered, planned actions with complete documentation (Action Implementation Planning Protocols), as presented in Figure 3.1.

DIRECT ACTION IMPLEMENTATION

As presented in Chapter 3, all actions from Level I observations can be implemented by the functional areas in which the observations were made. These actions are authorized by the functional areas, and action implementation is documented on the observation form (Exhibit 3.1). Action implementation records for Direct Action Implementation should include a description of the action, who implemented the action, date, time, and any anticipated impact. Actions identified from Level II/III observations may also be implemented through Direct Action Implementations after review by the Formal Investigation Team, without the need for a written action protocol. These actions include simple tasks and/or actions that have existing systems of control and traceability, e.g., document changes, product recalls/withdrawals, regulatory notifications, etc.

Action implementation, however, is not always a simple task. Consider the following:
- Some investigations identify many recommended actions that must be implemented in a coordinated manner to ensure the effectiveness of the actions.
- Some identified actions require action implementation across departments or divisions of the corporation.
- Some actions require complex implementation schedules, as plant or line shutdown and revalidations are required.
- Some actions require planning documents that are reviewed and approved by regulatory authorities.

In addition, once actions have been implemented, some actions require follow-up to assess their effectiveness, while some do not. As a result the other option for action implementation is to provide a tool for action planning, e.g. an Action Implementation Planning Protocol (AIPP), that details action implementation and effectiveness assessment requirements.

ACTION IMPLEMENTATION PLANNING

Action planning requires a comprehensive understanding of the actions to be implemented and the scheduling realities of operations, marketing, and/or regulatory review. Action planning must be executed in a manner that facilitates quick action but also accommodates adequate review of the plans. Action planning must include action effectiveness assessment plans, when appropriate, and the acceptance criteria for action effectiveness must be established in these controlled documents before the action is implemented.

Action implementation planning protocols. Action implementation planning protocols (AIPPs) provide the opportunity to detail action implementation/effectiveness assessment requirements, schedules, responsibilities, and acceptance criteria. These protocols also establish the results of risk-based decision making about when to assess effectiveness of actions, how much sampling is enough, how much testing, and what is statistically significant. These protocols need to be approved before action can begin. A form can be designed to facilitate the creation of a planning protocol. (Exhibit 6.1)

Action effectiveness failures. When the action effectiveness assessment is completed, either the action was effective or it was not effective. When actions are not effective it suggests that the "cause" of the problem, identified during the original investigation, may not have been the true cause. No matter what the reason, an ineffective action results in a continuing problem *and* in a change in a process or a product that is unnecessary. Ineffective actions should be eliminated from processes and products; eliminating them, however, is also a change that should be considered by the Action Analysis Team (Chapter 5).

Action failures are also observed when original problems recur. These recurring observations are detected during the investigative process, when the investigators perform retrospective review of other observations or investigations of similar problems.

ACTION TRACKING RECORDS, LOGS, AND NOTIFICATIONS

Action logs provide basic information about each action initiated from a Direct Action Authorization or each AIPP. The log facilitates tracking of progress from action identification to action implementation/effectiveness assessment closure. As discussed in Chapter 5, the timeliness of action implementation to correct problems is a regulatory expectation. Ensure that logs and records support timeliness requirements.

When Action Is Required Before the Investigation Is Complete

Although taking action before an investigation is complete is generally considered an unacceptable practice, there are occasions when action must be taken before the cause of the problem has been determined, e.g., regulatory notifications, equipment repairs, product disposition determinations, etc. As a result, provide a mechanism to identify these actions and highlight their associated investigations.

When action is taken before an investigation is conducted or completed, the rationale for that action must be documented and reviewed or approved by the Formal Investigation Team, and/or the Action Analysis Team. This is a risk-based decision and linking it to known risks identified for products (Chapter 1) or processes (as CCPs; Chapter 2) is important.

Actions Required by Regulatory Authorities for Distributed Products

All regulatory authorities have identified actions that must be taken when an event in the market and/or information from production and testing operations indicate that a patient or product user has been or could be hurt. The FDA has identified:

- FDA-requested product recalls in 21 CFR 7.45
- Firm-initiated product recalls in 21 CFR 7.46
- Corrections and removals for device products in 21 CFR 806
- Field alerts for drug products in 21 CFR 314.81
- Errors and accidents for biologic products in 21 CFR 600.14.

Other regulatory authorities and mutual recognition agreements between countries also require that authorities be notified of recalls, counterfeiting, and other quality problems that could require the suspension of product distribution in those countries. Regulatory Affairs in every company should identify all potential reporting requirements and ensure that the risk management framework facilitates an expedited analysis and review of these types of observations to ensure that reporting meets the requirements of regulatory authorities. Observations that require an action such as product recall, market withdrawal, or reports to regulatory authorities such as Errors and Accidents, Field Alerts, or Corrections and Removals should be Level III observations.

The reporting requirements associated with these types of observations are actions that may be taken before the investigation is complete. These types of actions, however, are not necessarily corrective actions, and an investigation to discover cause and determine corrective action must proceed.

Exhibit 6.1

Page __1__ of __1__

Action Implementation Planning Protocol

Action ID# _____

Describe the Action to be taken:
_____
_____

Preliminary operations before implementation _____
_____
_____

Who will implement? _____

When and how? _____
_____

What is considered an acceptable outcome of action? _____
_____

Who is responsible for information gathering and assessment? _____

When is assessment expected to be complete? _____

Action protocol written by _____ Date _____

Action effectiveness determination

Action implemented by _____ Date _____ Confirmed by _____ Date _____

Outcome ( ) meets the protocol requirements ( ) does not meet requirements

Reviewed by _____ Date _____

Attachments include _____

SECTION III

MANAGING FOR SAFETY AND PROFIT

CHAPTER 7

Why Things Go Wrong: Accident Theories in Innovative/Technologically Complex Industries

Most risk analysis, investigation, and corrective action procedures are designed to identify and eliminate known and potential accidents-of-design and accidents-of-procedure. There is, however, a third type of accident that haunts risk analysis and investigative teams; it lingers in Product Development and Operations like a disease that cannot be discussed. This is called an accident-of-management.

Executive management may be wary of the need to investigate or fix something that doesn't appear to be broken, especially when the company is profitable and compliant with regulatory expectations. But executive management also knows that one unexpected event can ruin a market opportunity and take down a company. No company wants to be an "industry example." Although delighted when a competitor begins to falter, company executives must realize that sometimes luck is involved.

One's fate, in the hands of the regulators or as a profitable, successful business, is not about luck. Problems in complex, technologically innovative industries are not impossible to solve, they are just different. They require better tools of analysis and investigation, more highly trained personnel, and management that is knowledgeable, responsive, and accountable for the resolution of technical problems. It is time to stop sweeping these difficult problems under the rug in the conference room and acknowledge the possibility that some of our technical problems are caused by accidents-of-management.

Types of Accidents

There are three types of accidents: accidents-of-procedure, accidents-of-design, and accidents-of-management.

Accidents-of-procedure are accidents that occur because mistakes are made and/or procedures are not followed. For example, test method controls fail because equipment has not been calibrated; a fermentation tank is contaminated because someone installed the wrong vent filter; a drug product fails to meet its potency specification because of a formulation error. These types of accidents can be avoided when technicians observe simple rules of procedure. Nevertheless, accidents-of-procedure will occur, and every regulated industry needs monitoring systems to assess ongoing compliance with existing procedures. (4)

Accidents-of-design are material, process, and product failures that should be predicted during design and validation but are not. For example:

- Babies are hurt because apnea monitors that monitor their breathing can be plugged directly into the power source; the monitoring leads are redesigned and the potential for the accident is eliminated.
- Twelve people die from polio after receiving the polio vaccine because the viral inactivation process is inadequate; the heat inactivation process is redesigned and the potential for infection eliminated.
- Serious latex sensitivity is observed in patients and clinicians; latex is removed from most products, warnings are placed on existing latex products, and the potential for reaction minimized.

Accidents-of-design, once discovered, can be eliminated or their impact minimized. The risk analysis processes of design controls (21 CFR 820.30), process validation (21 CFR 211.100), and clinical study help design engineers, development scientists, and clinicians detect and eliminate potential problems during product development, making accidents-of-design, once the product is in the market, less likely. Nevertheless, accidents-of-design will occur, and every regulated company needs monitoring systems to detect these problems; information from accidents-of-design should be used to redesign processes and products accordingly.

Those who investigate problems to determine cause in the complex world of medical product design, manufacture, testing, and use know that risk analysis and problem resolution are not simple tasks. Although procedures exist to detect and resolve accidents-of-procedure and accidents-of-design, there are other types of problems that are not easily understood or remedied. These are the problems that linger in outstanding investigations and corrective action backlogs; these are the problems that reappear long after corrective actions have been implemented.

Problems in complex technologies can also result when someone makes a faulty decision. Seldom is the cause of this type of accident or problem known immediately or conclusively. Although the procedures are followed to gather information, propose cause, honor regulatory deadlines and production schedules, and make more decisions, quick action to correct a problem takes precedence over the need to discover true cause; and seldom is the effectiveness of action measured or observed. In this decision-making environment, solutions for accidents-of-procedure and accidents-of-design are forced onto the record sheets of these investigations, and "technician error" becomes a common and recurring "cause" of problems. Nevertheless, there are standard procedures, they are followed, and the records are complete and compliant.

Although this approach, preventing and monitoring for accidents-of-procedure and accidents-of design, has been used for years in many medical product development/manufacturing companies, it is time to recognize that there is a third type of problem that occurs systematically: accidents-of-management. These accidents are not simple technical mistakes or simple personnel errors; they result from a combination of factors that have created an environment in which poor decision-making occurs, even with good people and sound technical data. Some schools of thought propose that these accidents occur because of inexperienced, inattentive, or inadequate management, and that the poor decision-making, which leads to the associated accident, could be controlled. Other schools of thought contend that these types of accidents are inevitable, that they are normal for our time, "science's illegitimate children . . . born of the confusion that lies with the complex organizations with which we manage our dangerous technologies." (4) Consider the following well-known examples:

- Valu-Jet Flight 592 takes off from Miami on a typical afternoon in May 1996 and within 10 minutes has crashed into the Everglades, killing all on board. Investigators discovered that Flight 592 was carrying oxygen canisters in the cargo; these canisters ignited and the resulting fire brought the plane down. Why were these canisters in the plane? Were they improperly labeled as "empty" by the canister rework contractor? Were the canisters improperly re-worked by the contractor, leaving the firing pins in tact? Were the canisters improperly loaded into the airplane? Were they improperly labeled by Valu-Jet as "airline parts" instead of hazardous materials? Was the inspection of the cargo hold by the supervisor and co-pilot, before take-off, inadequate? (4)
- The Space Shuttle Challenger explodes on January 26, 1986, because o-rings malfunctioned in the unusually cold air temperatures at the launch site that morning. How could engineers make the decision to

launch, knowing that the o-rings would not perform as intended at these temperatures? (1)
- In May 1996, twelve mountain climbers die from exposure on Mt. Everest. Many of the climbers died because they were on the mountain too late in the day. Decisions by expedition leaders allowing their clients to climb past the pre-determined "turn-around-times" ensured that more clients would reach the summit, but it also risked their lives. How could experienced leaders have made these decisions, in spite of weeks of intensive training about the importance of "turn-around-times"? (5)

All of these disasters occurred because individuals within these organizations made decisions that led to these mistakes, but the decisions themselves were "socially organized and systematically produced" by their respective organizations or corporations. These are not extraordinary organizations or extraordinary circumstances. Every organization develops a routine, taken-for-granted approach to business and decision making that creates a corporate "way-of-seeing" that is simultaneously a "way-of-not-seeing."(1) Most of the time, corporations get away with the little bad decisions that are inevitably made and things go right. But then one day a few bad decisions come together and the circumstances take down an airplane, a space shuttle, or a mountain climber. (4) Although all industries tend to blame these accidents on employee error, analysis in these investigations should have focused on why people made these particular decisions.

Some suggest that society simply accept the occasional disaster, because this is the added cost of complexity within innovative technologies. After all, dismantling any organization to fix or control all of these potential problems in decision making and management would ruin the business. Perhaps it is better to hire new management and hope "you get lucky". It is proposed, however, that when management in the medical products industry understands its role in the problem-solving process and is given the tools to manage risk, it can have a significant, positive impact on the day-to-day decision making that keeps a corporation well balanced between profitability and providing medical benefit to its market.

ACCIDENT THEORIES

In the study of accidents that have occurred in other regulated, hazardous technology industries, there are two perspectives on how to prevent accidents and maintain product safety. One perspective is the *High Reliability Theory* (2). This perspective maintains that with intelligent organizational design and management techniques a company can compensate for individual weaknesses within the organization and assure accident-free operations. The other perspective on accidents is developed from the *Normal Accident Theory* (2). This perspective maintains that serious accidents are inevitable. These theorists challenge many of the assumptions that support the High Reliability Theory. They have developed a perspective on organizational behavior that suggests that complex organizations make decisions in ways completely different from the rational models of the High Reliability theorists. This perspective reveals some of the more capricious aspects of organizational life that affect our ability to consistently produce safe products in a safe environment.

High Reliability Theory Perspective on Organizations

High Reliability theorists believe that there are four critical, causal factors that produce positive safety records within a wide variety of organizations: leadership that prioritizes safety objectives as an organizational goal, high levels of redundancy for product safety and essential personnel, a organizational culture of high reliability at the line level that is well-rehearsed, and a rigorous, organizational approach to trial-and-error learning. (2)

Leadership — One fundamental requirement for a high reliability organization is that reliability and safety must be a priority objective of executive management. Without this priority, money will not be spent to create the operational redundancies required to assure safety or to train staff adequately. Without clear and consistent communication of these priorities, the culture of safety and reliability that needs to reach to the line level in high-technology industries will not be achieved. (2)

Redundancy — Given the assumption that human beings do not perform perfectly or rationally every day, organizations have designed redundancies into their operations. High reliability organizations believe that multiple and independent channels of communication, production, testing and decision making can lead to greater reliability of the organization and the products as a whole, even if individual components of the organization or product are subject to error. Redundancy, implemented as duplication and overlap of technical and personnel resources, is a fundamental feature of operations in complex industrial processing. (2)

Decentralized Authority, Line Level Culture of Reliability, and Training — Redundant systems are designed for the problems that are deemed likely to occur. The success of redundant system design, therefore, depends on reducing the likelihood that the redundant systems will be needed. High Reliability organizations accomplish this by assuring a workforce that has:

- the authority and knowledge to react to problems when and where they occur

- the confidence to cope with unexpected events quickly and in a manner that supports product safety and reliability
- continuous experience and training that promotes vigilance and commitment. (2)

Trial-and-error Learning — Organizations must be designed to learn from their experiences, over time, and to adjust procedures and practices incrementally, to support the safety of their operations and their products.(2)

With the proper mix of organizational design and culture, the High Reliability theorists believe that safe operations and products can be assured.

NORMAL ACCIDENT THEORY PERSPECTIVE ON ORGANIZATIONS

Normal Accident theorists have examined the same industries as the High Reliability theorists, from a different perspective, and have concluded that "although complex organizations may work hard to maintain safety and reliability, serious accidents are nonetheless a "normal" result or an integral characteristic of the system." (2)

"Instead of clear and consistently communicated objectives, organizations operate on the basis of a variety of inconsistent and ill-defined preferences. Different individuals at different levels of the organization may hold conflicting goals . . . and although the organization manages to survive and even produce, its own processes are not understood by its members . . . the organizational left hand does not know what the right hand is doing . . . participants in the organizational decision-making processes come and go; some pay attention, while others do not; key meetings may be dominated by biased, uninformed or even uninterested personnel." (2)

The Normal Accident theorists have identified two characteristics of an industry that makes it susceptible to normal accidents: industries that display a high degree of interactive complexity and industries that are tightly coupled.

Industries with high interactive complexity have interdependent production processes that require many coordinated actions by numerous contractors, equipment systems, components, and operators. Despite years of experience, not every process is completely understood.

Tightly coupled industries have many time-dependent processes, and these processes must be performed without variation. Components and subassemblies must move through the production process in a pre-defined manner, and extensions and delays are not allowed. (2)

Medical product development and manufacturing industries qualify as both interactively complex and tightly coupled.

High Reliability vs. Normal Accidents

How does a Normal Accident theorist respond to the basic tenets of a High Reliability organization? (2)

Leadership — Normal Accident theorists agree that it is important for the company leaders to place a high priority on the objectives of safety and reliability, but there will continue to be conflict over goals. The pressure to maintain high production quotas or meet production schedules, for example, must be balanced against the safety agenda. Conflict with these other high-priority objectives can result in hasty decision making, shortcuts on safety, and special procedures.

Redundancy — Normal Accident theorists believe that adding redundancy to a system can increase the likelihood of failure. Designing redundant systems into a product or a process can increase the complexity of the system, which in turn increases the likelihood of common mode failures, and makes the system more difficult to understand. Finally, when systems or products are designed with multiple levels of redundancy, the perceived safety net can encourage the operators to move to higher or more dangerous levels of operation.

Decentralized Authority, Line Level Culture of Reliability, and Training — Although the Normal Accident theorists support the knowledgeable line worker, they also know that management seldom understands its technology, operations, or processes enough to determine how line level employees should respond to all contingencies. It is not possible to develop responses in advance of all unanticipated and undesirable failure modes in a highly interactive, tightly coupled industry.

Trial-and-error Learning — Although this is an admirable organizational goal, the reality is that effective learning is difficult. Causes of accidents are unclear; organizational leaders are likely to reconstruct the history of an event to support their own actions; reports of problems are biased to cover up errors; and secrecy between departments can make information gathering incomplete.

In summary, the High Reliability theorists believe that organizations can be designed and managed to near-perfect reliability and safety records. Normal Accident theorists believe that, in these same organizations, serious accidents are inevitable. The difference between these two schools of thought comes down to how much influence each one believes that management has on the performance of the organization. When management is informed and connected to the business of day-to-day risk assessment, problem analysis, and corrective action planning, it is capable of having a greater impact on product quality and business success. That impact, however, is not automatically positive.

ACCIDENTS-OF-MANAGEMENT

Accidents arise from the absence of knowledge at some point. Management is responsible for creating an environment in which information and people interact in a manner that focuses the social distribution of knowledge to assess risk and solve problems. In the environment of the Design Review Team in Product Development or the Formal Investigation Team in Operations, there are many common threats to good decision making. The following discussion addresses some of these threats.

NORMALIZATION OF DEVIANCE

"Part of the effectiveness of organizations lies in the way they are able to bring together large numbers of people and imbue them for a sufficient time with a sufficient similarity of approach, outlook and priorities to enable them to achieve collective, sustained responses which would be impossible if a group of unorganized individuals were to face similar problems. However, this very property also brings with it the dangers of a collective blindness to important issues, the danger that some vital factors may be left outside the bounds of organizational perception.

"When a pervasive and structural set of beliefs bias . . . an organization and its members, these beliefs do not merely show up in the attitudes and perceptions of the men and women within the organization, but they also affect the decision-making procedures." (6)

When managers successfully develop a cohesive and communicative group of people with expertise and experience in risk assessment and problem solving, it is tempting to believe that the work of management is done. It is not. Groups can learn to accept deviant observations as normal because of a variety of environmental influences.

- Group thinking can discourage learning from experience. Data that conflict with prior decisions and actions can be easily rejected from the group. Similarly, individuals who challenge the group's interpretation are often minimized with statements like, "you just don't understand how we work around here."
- Groups can expand the definition of "normal" incrementally, over time. As long as things go right, it is considered acceptable; with enough time, what was once considered an unacceptable risk becomes accceptable.
- Group success can bias a group to take more risks or shortcuts, relying on what they think they know rather than what they know through data derived from testing and observation.
- Group success can result in group arrogance, fostering a belief that they know when a product is "OK," even if the data indicate otherwise.

- Groups can collectively promote an institutionalization of solutions to problems such as "worker error" or "cause unknown" if group success is judged by the quantity of work or its timeliness, rather than the effectiveness of work.
- Management can bias group performance with:
  - predetermined outcomes, often communicated in the way a problem is presented
  - timelines that favor only certain conclusions
  - unplanned or project-specific changes in team membership, configuration, or leadership
  - prioritization of business success over technical discovery.

Consider the following example of the "normalization of deviance," taken from an FDA warning letter in 1998.

"During the validation process the following occurred: in the first set of biological challenge runs, six out of seven runs were positive for growth. . . . the positive growth was attributed to problems with the inoculation procedure. . . . during the second set of runs, two out of seven runs were positive for growth. The positive growth was attributed to the high jacket pressure of the autoclave. The third set of runs were made with adjustments to the jacket pressure. One out of five runs was positive for growth. After an inconclusive investigation, one additional run was made and no growth was found. It was concluded . . . that the process is validated. None of the initial three sets of runs met the acceptance criteria outlined in the validation protocol. . . ."

INFORMATION REPORTING VARIABLES

"In story books — and undoubtedly still in some graduate courses in basic management practices — the true condition is easy to describe. Challenges arrive sequentially. Information is gathered. Wise heads are consulted. A plan is formed. Contingencies are pondered and provided for. Ducks are lined up. The big guns are pulled out. And finally a solution is executed.

"In the real world nothing happens like that. In the real work billions of variables interact continuously. In the real world, if you study all the information available . . . you might go blind from reading. There is too much of it and . . . it is too instantaneously accessible." (7)

Controlling the quality, quantity, and flow of information to risk-based decision-making groups is essential to success. There are many aspects of information gathering, information organization/analysis, and information reporting/presentation that can affect how the information is used.

- Some people respond to data when it is heard; some people respond to data when it is seen; some people respond to data when it is presented

by another person, face-to-face. The format and configuration of data presentation can have a significant impact on the social distribution of the information to those most likely to contribute to the problem solving process.
- All information is biased by the individuals collecting it, reviewing it, and presenting it. When data is presented, it is important to know data origin.
- Data gathering is easily biased to:
  – be self-serving, reinforcing previous conclusions or theories,
  – confirm what management wants or is likely to support.
- Data gathering can be compromised by products and systems that are too complex to master or test completely. The need for specialized knowledge to understand data increases a sense of powerlessness about its usefulness; and people will rely on what they *think* they know rather than what they know in the face of this confusion.
- Data acceptability is often influenced by the individuals presenting the data. If the individual is not a socially accepted member of the group, their data may be ignored, no matter what its impact.
- Getting good information requires wanting it and using it. When information sources find that their information is seldom acknowledged or seldom used in associated analysis, they can falter in the rigor of their effort to produce reliable, accurate data and observations.
- Faulty reporting of information is inevitable when it is not in the best interests of the operator to acknowledge the existence of mistakes, problems, or accidents. Secrecy about information/data can be in the personal self-interest of the worker, sometimes even in the self-interest of the group or department.

Summit fever

In the environment of a start-up, entrepreneurial company, there must be a belief that the overly demanding and optimistic goals of the company can be achieved. These companies are filled with individuals who are betting their careers on the likelihood that they can beat the odds. This is a very self-motivated group of individuals, aligned together toward a common mission. It is a group that is not likely to take bad news or unexpected data at face value. There is always resistance, a tendency to disregard the information, deny its value, or challenge the messenger. This group attitude is, as a result, always a challenge for those performing design reviews and risk analysis of new products.

Blue Goo . . . "was the company's lead product. In 1992, after an early round of trials, the company reported that Blue Goo seemed effective in healing nasty wounds on the feet of diabetic patients who otherwise faced amputation. . . . [B]ut last October . . . the drug failed to outperform a placebo in its definitive Phase III clinical trial . . . within minutes . . . stock fell 68%. . . . [T]here were warning signs that . . . early analysis of experimental data was unsound. And some shareholders allege that the data were deliberately manipulated to mask shortcomings and keep the product alive. Clinical trial experts say, there is little mystery . . . the company engaged in data dredging, dismissing the overall — and unfavorable — results of what it set out to prove . . . and focusing on apparent success among a handful of trial participants." (8)

Similarly, in the environment of commercial manufacturing, production schedules and profitability are minimum expectations of performance. Production pressures can make management blind to problems. The following events are not fictitious.
- Product specifications are changed after the product is produced, so that a previously unacceptable product becomes acceptable.
- Unacceptable bulk product is mixed into acceptable bulk product, tested to meet specification, and released as acceptable.
- A product failure is considered acceptable because an investigation was performed as directed in an SOP, and the paperwork is done.
- The investigation of a process failure is considered complete and acceptable when the technician has been reprimanded, retrained, or reassigned.

CRISIS AND STRESS

Crisis does not bring out the best in people, it brings out the creativity. Crisis situations create stressful work environments, and workers will take shortcuts to meet demands. Under the stress of market approval, or production schedules, when someone skips a step or does not follow the rules for the higher good of the organization, misconduct becomes organizationally "OK." Stress and production pressures can compromise the performance of risk-based decision-making groups and change the quality of the decisions that they make.

MANAGEMENT IS RESPONSIBLE FOR THE DECISION-MAKING ENVIRONMENT

Management is responsible for maintaining a decision-making environment that supports efficient and effective risk and problem analysis. This environment is not simply established by standard operating procedures; it is also defined by a complex social interaction of people interacting with data to make decisions, i.e., the socio-technical interface. As suggested earlier, there are those who have studied other high-technology organizations in regulated industries who believe that the socio-technical interface can be controlled. They have suggested control points in the organization that have positive impact, and risk-based decision-making processes should be designed with these controls in place. Nevertheless, as the Normal Accident theorists remind us, control is never complete, and management must be vigilant.

When management provides and maintains a healthy, risk-based decision-making environment, as presented in Chapter 8, the balance between profits and product safety can be maintained and the surprises posed by accidents-of-design and accidents-of-procedure can be minimized.

CITED REFERENCES

1. Vaughn, Diane. 1996. *The Challenger Launch Decision*. Chicago: University of Chicago Press.
2. Sagan, Scott D. 1993. *Limits of Safety*. Princeton, NJ: Princeton University Press.
3. Perrow, Charles. 1984. *Normal Accidents: Living with High Risk Technologies*. New York: Basic Books.
4. Langewiesche, William. 1998. "The Lessons of Valu-Jet 592." *Atlantic Monthly* (March).
5. Krakauer, Jon. 1997. *Into Thin Air*. New York: Villard Books.
6. Turner, B. A., and N. F. Pidgeon. 1997. *Man-Made Disasters*. Oxford: Butterworth-Heinemann.
7. Taylor, James, and Watts Wacker. 1997. *The 500 Year Delta*. New York: HarperCollins.
8. King, Jr., Ralph T. 1994. "A Tale of a Dream: A Drug and Data Dredging." *Wall Street Journal* (February 7, 1994).

REFERENCES

More, Thomas J. 1995. *Deadly Medicine*. New York: Simon and Schuster.

Pool, Robert. 1997. *Beyond Engineering*. New York: Oxford University Press.

Reason, James. 1999. *Managing Risks of Organizational Accidents*. Brookfield, VT: Ashgate Publishing Company.

Weinberg, Robert A. 1997. *Racing to the Beginning of the Road*. New York: Harmony Books.

CHAPTER 8

MANAGING RISK-BASED DECISION-MAKING GROUPS TO PROTECT PROFITS AND PRODUCT SAFETY

Risk-based decision-making groups act like an immune system for the corporation. They protect a project, a product, or a facility from potential problems; and they mitigate the adverse impact of real problems on a daily basis. A human being is protected by two types of immunity. The first defense roams throughout the body to provide an efficient and effective response at the point of injury or infection. The second line of defense is located in specialized organ systems like the lymph systems and spleen where, when warranted, a more orderly and comprehensive attack can be launched. Similarly, a corporation depends on two lines of defense. The first defense lies in the individual actions of every employee to do his or her job, as directed, and solve potential problems (accidents-of-procedure and accidents-of-design) before they become real problems. The second line of defense is provided by specialized groups of people, trained to detect and solve difficult problems that could threaten the health of the corporation.

Managing groups that make risk-based decisions requires an uncommon level of responsible leadership. Although establishing good hazard identification and risk analysis procedures (as discussed in Section I) may initially satisfy regulators, it is the ongoing performance of the risk-based decision makers and their use of risk analysis reports that has the greatest impact on business performance. Just as an incompetent immune system can threaten one's life, a poorly managed risk-based decision-making group can threaten the life of the corporation either by its inadequate performance, leaving the corporation defenseless, or by its overzealousness, leading to the corporate equivalent of an autoimmune disease.

Each company, depending on its market and its business mission, will have a variable mix of these groups (examples provided in Section II). There are, nevertheless, points to consider in their performance and organization (Chapter 9) that can significantly impact their effectiveness:

1) Segregation of Technical Risk-Based Decision Makers from Business Risk-Based Decision Makers
2) Rigorous Group Organization, Training, and Monitoring
3) Decision-Making Meeting Controls
4) Leadership from Executive Management

1) Segregation of Technical Risk-Based Decision Makers from Business Risk-Based Decision Makers

The performance of a risk-based decision-making group is enhanced when their mission is defined and focused by one set of corporate values. As discussed in Chapter 5, a technical risk-based decision-making group, for example the group responsible for formal investigations, is likely to falter when asked to simultaneously balance technical risk with business risk. A dominant business culture and its associated values can erode a technical culture, leading to an ever-increasing number of unresolved technical problems. Similarly, a dominant technical culture can erode the business culture, leading to an ever-increasing cost of innovation and compliance. Either one of these biases will impact profitability. **Segregate technical risk-based decisions from business risk-based decisions, as presented in Chapter 5, and always conduct business risk decision-making *after* technical evaluations have been completed and actions proposed.**

Symptoms of business culture dominance are more visible to independent observers; nevertheless, a retrospective internal review of decision making can identify this potential problem before it becomes a regulatory risk. The risk-based decision-making groups have failed the corporation because of business culture dominance when regulatory risks are evident, for example, when:

- drug product is released to the market after failing five out of six potency determinations
- product is released to the market after failing two out of three sterility tests
- product is left in distribution when stability/shelf life data indicates that its "use before" date is not valid

- a definitive, Phase III, 30 center, $10 million study is launched and a $4.5 million facility is built after only seven out of twenty-eight patients benefited from treatment, less than the control.

Symptoms of business culture dominance

When it is suspected that business culture dominance is compromising the effectiveness of group performance, look for the following common patterns of biased performance:

- Technical risk-based decisions, although rigorously developed, are routinely ignored and overruled by management decisions.

    Technical risk-based decision making, e.g., product risk analysis (Chapter 1), process hazard identification (Chapter 2), or Formal Investigation (Chapter 5), is rigorous, time-consuming work. When that work is not valued, or when the decisions of the group are continually overruled by Management decisions, the group becomes demoralized. Work shifts from doing good problem analysis to pushing the paperwork through the system. Work shifts from determination of true cause to justification of management's predetermined decisions.

- Technical risk-based decisions that are inadequate or incomplete because the success of the group is not measured in technical terms or accomplishments. There is no reward, either monetary or sociological, for good, technical, risk-based decision-making.

    Underlying the Challenger Launch decision of 1986, for example, was a program whose success, year after year, was judged on the basis of economics rather than ongoing engineering achievements. As a result, "competition, scarce resources, and production pressures . . . were the structural origins of the disaster. They permeated the NASA organization, affecting decision-making on the eve of launch. Far from being incompetent, those responsible for the decision to launch were experienced managers who understood thoroughly both the technical and managerial issues involved. Understanding, they made a choice." (1)

- Technical risk-based decisions that are inadequate or incomplete because the problems are framed by management before the investigations are conducted. All information gathering is biased, in that information is gathered only to justify predetermined business decisions.

    Engineers at NASA were asked, in the decision-making associated with the Challenger Launch of 1986, to shift their information gathering and analysis process from demonstrating that the o-rings would work to proving that they would not work. Instead of determining risk, they were asked to justify decision making. What may seem like a subtle shift in focus can cripple the information gathering and analysis process. (1)

2) Risk-Based Decision-Making Group Organization, Performance, Training, and Monitoring

The technical analysis and problem solving required to assure the consistent quality of medical products requires a multidisciplinary approach. Without participation from a variety of functional area experts, determining the cause of problems and developing reasonable options for corrective action will be compromised by short-sighted vision.

Do not assign group participants based solely on ranking or position in the corporation; pick individuals with expertise *and* with an open-minded approach to work and problems. Group members should:

- be technically knowledgeable about the work and the work environment of medical product development, manufacturing, testing, and distribution
- have convenient access to the associated facilities and the individuals who routinely perform the work
- be welcomed and comfortable in these areas or facilities, as their ability to ask questions and get honest answers is fundamental to their success as troubleshooters.

The more information available to characterize a problem, the more likely that proposed cause will be the true cause and that corrective actions will be effective.

Good group performance requires:
- a clear, focused mission of the group
- established processes for work input, work flow, work conduct, and work output
- specialized training and development
- established integration of information with other risk-based decision-making groups.

Establish a clear, focused mission for the group

A risk-based decision-making group consists of people that interact because they have a common task. Groups are well organized when the expertise of individual members is focused on certain types of problems or risks. This is the basis for the recommendation to separate business risk decision makers from technical risk decision makers, discussed in Chapter 5. Similar advantage can be gained in separating market risk-based decision making, which relies on those knowledgeable about external consumers, clinicians, product users, and user environments, from technical risk-based decision making, which relies on those knowledgeable about the technical attributes of the products and internal manufacturing/testing environments.

With the mission of the group established, the numbers and types of individuals appropriate for group membership can be determined. Some groups, in particular those designated for Design Review according to 21 CFR 820.30 (e), require an objective, third-party member of the review team. When developing any group, consider training an independent consultant or another participant that can be brought into the group on request.

Establish work input, work flow, work conduct, and output criteria

Systematic processing of data and observations is required for hazard identification, risk analysis, Formal Investigation, and corrective/preventive action implementation planning. Each systematic process should be established in writing and followed. In addition, risk-based decision-making groups also benefit from establishing minimum requirements for work input. Just as FDA review has benefited from "refuse to file" policy, groups require a minimum amount of information, team member participation, etc., before the analysis process can be initiated. Without these requirements specified, the group can be vulnerable to the influences of tribal rituals based primarily on the dominance of personalities and organizational culture rather than on good objective analysis.

Train and develop risk-based decision-making groups

Every risk-based decision-making group should be established (defined, documented, and implemented) and trained for performance. Management should invest in specialized training for the group to develop hazard identification, risk analysis, and investigative skills. In addition Management should invest in developing a well-rehearsed group culture that will promote mutual respect and trust among group members, an essential characteristic in groups where confrontation and conflict are the tools of decision making.

"Construct decision-making teams and procedures for intensive problem solving before they are needed. . . . in order to make basically one hundred percent correct decisions in extremely short periods of time . . . you learn to communicate and assess data, you learn to make reasonably crisp and authoritative decisions, you learn to admit when you don't know what's going on and ask for help." (2)

Group members must be given the specialized tools to do their work, and they must learn to use these tools as a team. Develop group dynamics that optimize the performance of the group over its individual members. Group members must be willing to give time, actively participate in group decision making, and be responsible for the group's work. In addition, group members must establish the trust and mutual respect needed to survive the conflict essential to good, risk-based decision making.

Specialized tools of risk-based decision making include:
- hazard identification
- risk analysis
- investigation techniques
- information analysis and triage
- decision making
- action planning
- confrontation and conflict as allies in the negotiation of risk.

In addition, consider the need to identify and/or develop human resources for these groups before they are needed. Identify and train:
- specialized knowledge experts
- backup team members
- independent leadership for difficult or crisis situations
- conflict resolution experts.

Identify training and development criteria for the group such as: introduction of new members, new product updates, new technology updates, and periodic retraining and development to facilitate changes in procedure, work flows, and group dynamics.

Integrate information between risk-based decision-making groups

Although every risk-based decision-making group is responsible for a multidisciplinary approach to problems, their perspective is biased by a common set of values, e.g., technical, business, or market. To maintain the profitability of the company and the safety of the consumer, all of these perspectives and their associated value systems must be balanced. Consider the need to integrate information between all groups that determine risk or make risk-based decisions.

Risk-Based Decision-Making Groups in Product Development. This group bases its decision making on a value system that emphasizes the product design; hazards are identified as those things likely to compromise product safety, performance, or ability to meet its intended use. Risks are calculated from knowledge about:

- the technical design features of the product and its associated manufacturing processes (Section I)
- the user, the user environment and the market (Chapters 1, 4).

The output of product risk analysis or process hazard identification is provided to ongoing operations to facilitate a risk-based approach to problem identification and triage. Product Development, however, should remain connected to the risk-based decision-making groups, as new hazards are identified and risk levels redefined during routine use of the product.

Formal Investigation Team in Operations. The Formal Investigation Team is responsible for responding to serious problems discovered during routine operations in commercial manufacturing, testing, and distribution of products. The Formal Investigation Team must segregate technical risk-based decisions from business risk-based decisions, conclude technical risk-based investigations and action proposals before the business risks are considered, and then authorize action (Chapters 5, 6).

Action Analysis Team in Operations. This team supports the Formal Investigation Team in Operations. They review actions proposed to solve the most serious problems (Level III and some Level II observations from Chapter 3) for their business impact. Utilizing business risk-based decision making to edit and audit the technical risk-based decisions allows for balance between product safety and corporate profit objectives (Chapter 5).

Complaint/Adverse Event Management Groups. This group bases its decision making on a value system that emphasizes the risks associated with the patient, the consumer/user, or the market. This group monitors the market and the user environment for complaints and adverse events associated with product use, which may provide valuable information about product performance. Serious complaints or adverse events must be investigated and often reported to regulatory authorities. Determining the seriousness of an event is based on the Product Risk Analysis Report and process hazard identification.

MONITOR AND CONTROL OF GROUP PERFORMANCE

Group performance is threatened by many aspects of organizational life that have been established over time. Consider the following threats to performance:
- normalization of deviance
- inadequate procedures
- inadequate group performance in spite of good procedures
- group dominance by individuals
- overconfidence.

Normalization of deviance. "The explanation of the Challenger launch is a story of how people who work together develop patterns that blind them to the consequences of their actions. It is not only about the development of norms but about the incremental expansion of normative boundaries: how small changes — new behaviors that are slight deviations from the normal course of events — gradually became the norm, providing a basis for accepting additional deviance. No rules are violated; there is no intent to do harm . . . it is a story that illustrates how disastrous consequences can emerge from the banality of organizational life." (1)

Normalization of deviance relies on the opposite of Murphy's Law; if something can go wrong, it usually doesn't. With enough time and experience, what was once considered a risk or a deviation becomes acceptable, and then new risks are taken. Incrementally, experience is substituted for rigorous analysis, and high risks become acceptable risks. Change is made and more risk is taken without the benefit of new risk analysis . . . until one day Murphy returns. (3)

Medical products are sometimes released into the marketplace when they have failed to meet established, final product specifications. The organizational rationale behind such a decision is, usually, "but we know the product is good; we can't prove it yet, but we just know its good; it has always been good before." This is how deviance is normalized: accept the deviance once, suffer no adverse consequences, and soon this behavior can become acceptable, organizational practice, no matter how risky the practice from a regulatory perspective. (Consult Chapter 7.)

Inadequate procedures. Risk-based decision-making groups do not follow procedure when the procedure is inadequate. Procedures are inadequate when:
- they are not clearly written
- they are not understood by those performing the work that they describe
- there is little time to do the work required
- the work that they demand seems useless to the user.

Assuming that procedures are not followed because "trained workers need more training" can be a shortsighted fix to a bigger problem. If not following procedures is an issue for your groups, be prepared to redesign work flow, rewrite procedures and reconsider the value of the tasks that are required.

Inadequate group performance in spite of good procedures: Many organizations have acceptable procedures for risk-based decision making that are followed. Problems are discovered, they are investigated, actions are taken, the paperwork is flawless, and there are no outstanding issues. The fact that procedures are followed, however, does not mean that a good investigation or good risk analysis is performed. Group performance must be measured appropriately. Did the investigation discover cause, for example? Did the implemented corrective actions solve the problem? Do problems recur?

Group dominance by individuals. Risk-based decision-making groups rely on multidisciplinary interactions for success. As a result, when the group is dominated by one individual, group performance is compromised. This condition may arise because of a dominant personality, or it may arise because other group members are not willing or not allowed to devote adequate time to their risk management responsibilities.

Use of outside consultants to lead group discussion can refocus group dynamics, but outsiders can also bias the group toward management concerns or objectives when the observer is sent by management. As suggested earlier, it is good practice for a group to identify someone to work with the group, upon request, who knows the rules of conduct, the products, and the group mission. Rotation of group leadership, internally within the group, also facilitates lack of domination. This allows everyone the opportunity to direct the risk management process, and can promote adherence to procedures while maintaining undominated group participation.

Overconfidence. When the group rejects conflicting information quickly or rejects anyone who does not agree with their perspective of the problems at hand, group success is threatened by overconfidence and a false sense of objectivity. Overconfidence can restrict information flow and information analysis. Independent group leadership can minimize this threat.

3) Decision-Making Meeting Controls

Good risk-based decision-making groups identify problems quickly and solve them proactively by focusing the social distribution of knowledge about a hazard or a problem. Acceptable risk is a social negotiation, and social negotiation is influenced by the performance environment in which problems are considered.

Decision-making meetings benefit from establishing:
- agenda consistency
- planning, notification, and meeting preparation requirements
- minimum requirements for information quality and presentation
- rules of conduct
- rules for decision making
- consistent group leadership.

Agenda consistency

Run every meeting according to a consistent agenda. This offers reliability of information flow and, with time and practice, it provides a predictable structure in which participants can offer their input and know when their opinions will be solicited. Typical agenda items for decision-making groups include:

- assess progress against plans from previous meetings
- present and/or analyze new problems
- identify decisions to make
- make decisions
- initiate new action plans
- revise existing plans
- identify new work assignments
- designate next meeting.

Meeting notification and preparation requirements

Establish meeting notification requirements, even if the meetings are, predictably, every Thursday. The notification event can remind meeting participants to read premeeting information packages. Every active, voting member of the group must read the information package *before* the meeting begins.

Since most meetings require data review, ensure that all information is available in written form and distributed for review before the meeting. Discourage data package surprises or last-minute presentations of new material. Decision making based on last-minute data, under the pressure of group dynamics, is not an acceptable, standard practice. Individuals reviewing written information in the privacy of their offices provide a different and very valuable assessment process that is lost if information is reviewed only in a group setting. Prereview also provides time for group members to seek supporting information that facilitates group discussion.

Information quality, analysis, and presentation requirements

Although data must be clear, concise, relevant, and consistently communicated, not everyone responds to or understands data the same way. Some are more comfortable with data presented in written form; some understand only concepts and problems that are presented visually. When presenting data to a group, require it in written form and as an oral presentation with visual aids, even if the visual aid is simply the written data projected on a screen in the meeting room.

Establish and follow rules for the production and exchange of data. Train all participants to clearly identify the difference between what they know, when it is supported by evidence, and what they think they know, when probabilities are involved. When untrained participants present to the group, this clarification is essential to true understanding of data, summaries, and opinions. Train all participants to clearly identify the source of all data, because knowing who produced the data can be beneficial to understanding what weight to give it in the decision-making process.

Rules of conduct

Information analysis is about making connections; groups must establish rules of presentation that maximize the ability to connect data, information, and observations to solve problems. Establish rules of conduct for meeting discussions that will help to create an environment that encourages the exchange of ideas and information. Consider the following aspects of group conduct:

- Hierarchies that exist outside the group can be carried over to compromise open and full participation. Establish rules to minimize the impact of such hierarchies; managers, line workers and development scientists must enjoy equivalent status within the group.
- Configure all critical meetings as face-to-face discussions. In this age of videoconferencing and conference calls, understanding complex information can be compromised when the body language and inflection of the presenter are hidden from view.
- Create an environment in which people want to cooperate and solve problems, but do not confuse calmness and friendliness with cooperation; controversy is what gets problems solved! Create an environment in which members feel safe challenging one another or the data presented.
- Talk is what helps a group sort complex issues and arrive at multiple options. "Acceptable risk" is a social negotiation and risk-based decision making groups must consider the perspectives of all disciplines to bring confidence to their decision making. Develop rules to encourage participation from all members.
- Provide a mechanism for the group to pause, reconsider, and reconvene; provide any group member the opportunity to stop a decision-making process without retribution.

Rules for decision making

The decision-making process of a group should be defined before the information is gathered and analyzed, and the decision making must be performed as directed. If voting is fundamental to the process, anticipate what happens when members are absent, when there is a stalemate, etc. When information or problems have been classified according to levels of risk, the decision-making process may vary according to the type of risk.

Do not let anyone, especially management, change this decision-making process for special cases. Establish the process; follow the process.

There are patterns of human nature evident in the decision-making process that can bias outcomes, even when procedures are followed. Consider the following:

- The mind will give disproportionate weight to the first information it receives.

- There is always a strong bias toward answers or solutions that preserve the status quo, i.e., "let's not rock the boat."
- Choices are preferred that justify past choices, even when those choices no longer seem valid, i.e., "throwing good money after bad."
- We seek information that supports our view and do not seek information that opposes our view.
- People are risk averse when problems are posed in terms of gains; people are risk seeking when problems are posed in terms of avoiding loss (4).

Group leadership

Group leaders are responsible for monitoring the effectiveness of individual participants in the group and assuring the success of the group's performance, technically, as defined by executive management. Group leaders are responsible for creating and maintaining an environment in which good decisions can be made by the group. When possible, group leaders should not be voting members of the group in the decision-making processes.

4) Leadership from Management

Be an advocate for risk-based decision making

Managing risk-based decision-making groups requires vigilant advocacy with executive management to maintain the resources required for their effective performance. Because these groups are asked to focus on the weaknesses of the operation, executive management seldom solicits information about their performance, and if things are going well, they are invisible. Executive management is usually aware of risk management activities only when something has gone wrong. As a result, when budgets are tight, it is easy to cut the resources supporting these groups.

Responsible group managers must understand the value of risk analysis as a basic building block of good business practice. With this understanding, they must remain advocates for risk-based decision making in the hard times and recover resources when times are good. In Product Development, for example, cost constraints may result in decreased safety testing of components, or less risk analysis after a product design is complete. Each of these potential actions will cripple troubleshooting about that product for years to come. It is, in reality, a "pay now or pay later" proposition, and yet it is one that the business culture of a start-up company finds very clear: "there won't be a 'later' if we don't get market approval." Market authorization and market success do not indicate that a product is risk-free. Remember, it is the opposite of Murphy's Law—"if it can go wrong, it usually doesn't"—and you can be lulled into a false sense of safety without a safety net.

Accept conflict and confrontation as essential to risk-based decision making

Management wants cooperation and control, and yet good risk-based decision making requires confrontation and conflict. Management is expected to develop and maintain a system of cooperation in their respective departments and/or facilities, to motivate employees and to formulate organizational objectives. This, by necessity, relegates the real work of research, development, manufacturing, testing, and marketing to another level of worker. As a result, a barrier emerges between the real work and the organizational processes that can make management of risk-based decision makers unique, if not difficult. (5)

Bureaucracies, after all, reward those who fit in, those who align with the corporate ideal, those who avoid blame, those who protect their own, those who have allies. Although bureaucracies depend on them, they do not commonly reward those who stand by their actions or those who perceive errors in their products or processes.

It is no wonder that those charged with managing risk in the corporation are often perceived as negative personalities by executive management. When they are good at what they do, they perceive errors, challenge existing practices, stand up for what they know, and act without respect for hierarchy or the need for allies. It is human nature to blame the messenger when the message is negative or the message does not support the worldview that the corporation might have of itself.

Management must allow risk-based decision-making groups to probe and pick at the company's established operations and worldview, understanding that this monitoring and control function is helping to ensure strength. It may be uncomfortable, but it can keep that canary alive in the coal mine.

Avoid cultures of blame

There is a significant difference between a culture-of-responsibility and a culture-of-blame. In a culture-of-responsibility, individuals are expected to be responsible for the work they do, to act on behalf of the organization in their decision making, and to notify superiors when they do not understand something or observe something unexpected. If at any time in the history of the corporation, however, there has been a "culture-of-blame," in which individuals are systematically blamed, demoted, or fired for mistakes or problems, it is very difficult to manage risk. Blame cultures foster secrecy; secrecy can inhibit information gathering; and without reliable information, problems remain unsolved.

In industries that do not require high technology workers, a culture-of-blame is common; this culture is from a former industrial era when worker input was not considered valuable to management. In high technology industries, however, workers are highly educated and their input is vital to product quality. It is the tendency of an educated worker to blame himself when something goes wrong. In industries that have attempted to make the transition from low tech to high tech, the residual cultures can sabotage good troubleshooting and risk management (Chapter 9).

KNOW WHEN TO SEIZE AUTHORITY AND WHEN TO LET GO

Organizations are created to focus the energies of a large number of individuals, representing various disciplines, on a single problem. This requires that the organization and its associated rules of conduct be centralized, i.e., dictated by executive management.

Once created, however, management in high-technology industries must also establish decentralized authority, i.e., the authority to act independently at lower levels of the hierarchy, when crisis demands action. Decentralized authority requires established, open lines of communication that travel *up* the hierarchy of the organization (opposite the lines of communication established in centralized-authority organizations). (Consult Chapters 7 and 9.)

This two-tiered approach to management balances centralized and decentralized authority to the benefit of the organization. The organization must be structured to both (a) *provide* information that everyone needs to work together and (b) *receive* information from the "front lines," i.e. the engineers, scientists, technicians, salespeople, and line workers that interact with the technology, on a daily basis (Chapter 9). These individuals are the "eyes and ears" of the corporation. They are the individuals most likely to see potential problems before they occur, and most likely to know the effectiveness of actions taken.

These lines of communication, however, must be established and individuals trained in these authorities. With consistent training in the purpose and goals of the organization, the rules of hierarchy can be de-emphasized. This approach requires a strong understanding of who can do what (individual capabilities) and how power is balanced. If authority is left to goodwill, it will become unbalanced. Identify decision points, and educate for the mission of the whole and the responsibilities of individuals.

The ability to create organizations that provide for both centralized and decentralized authority, depending on the circumstances, is more commonly an American construct. This is important to realize and appreciate, especially in this era of multinational organizations. Americans want and expect a high-technology workforce to be thinking human beings, not puppets, because they depend on them to provide both the discipline required to develop, manufacture, and test medical products and the confidence required to know what to do when things do not go as planned. (8, 9)

Consider the cultural influences beyond the corporation

Although Americans believe that the flexibility offered by a balance between centralized and decentralized authorities is organizationally beneficial and responsible for America's innovation and entrepreneurial success, not every culture embraces the benefits of flexibility. Balancing different management styles in the workplace, which arrive with managers from different ethnic and corporate cultures, is a company-specific challenge.

No matter what the organizational style of management, however, risk-based decision-making groups operate more effectively as a group without hierarchy inside the group. If the group's style is compatible with corporate management styles, then the group will have convenient access to information from other functional areas of the corporation to enhance its capabilities and performance. When access to information is blocked by corporate structures/cultures outside of the group, information may be biased by the communication channel it must navigate, and group performance is compromised. Management can seldom eliminate these barriers, but if it is aware of these issues, it can take action to minimize their impact on the success of the risk-based decision-making processes.

Provide confidence and optimism

Management is responsible for maintaining the optimism so essential to focused, rigorous work with ever-changing variables. Management must believe in the success of the group and be an advocate for them when their resources are threatened. The famous line of Eugene Kranz paraphrased in the Ron Howard movie *Apollo 13*, "Failure is not an option," is not a product of blind optimism but of trained confidence (2). Management's expectation of high performance is a prerequisite to its achievement by the workers, and yet overconfidence on the part of management can become "summit fever" (Chapter 7).

Stay connected

High-technology work requires a strong connection between management and workers to build influence through trust and empathy as much as power and control. Management must stay connected to risk-based decision-making groups in order to assure the adequacy of their work loads, resources, and performance. Management must stay connected to know about their successes and progress, firsthand. Do not allow this connection, however, to influence the outcome of their decision-making processes.

Monitor group performance

Regulatory authorities expect management to monitor the performance of its quality systems. This is an FDA expectation (21CFR 820.20 (c)):

"Management with executive responsibility shall review the suitability and effectiveness of the quality system at defined intervals and with sufficient frequency according to established procedures to ensure that the quality system satisfies the . . . objectives." This is also an ISO 9004 expectation: "The management with executive responsibility should . . . carry out periodic reviews of the quality results."

For risk-based decision-making groups, this expectation is not satisfied with the self-audits. "One should never assume that the machine does not need to be fixed, simply because one has been told that it ain't broke." (7) When the "machine" is human performance, reporting on group performance by well-bonded group members is likely biased to protect the reputation of the group. Monitor group performance with independent auditors. Look for:

- trends in decision making
- recurring problems
- new problems related to previous problems or actions
- incomplete or inadequate analysis of change or deviation
- lack of time to prevent problems.

Trends in Decision Making. Look for trends in decision making; look for common causes of problems, common solutions to problems, and trends of success. As suggested numerous times throughout this text, there are some organizational threats that only an outsider can see. Groups that function seamlessly, with little conflict, may be vulnerable to the negative effects of group culture, i.e., the normalization of deviance.

Recurring Problems. Look for the frequency of similar problems. This can indicate the inadequacy of actions, the failure to determine the true cause of a deviation, or incomplete analysis of problems for associated potential problems.

New Problems. Evaluate newly identified problems for any association to previous actions. When corrective actions are implemented, new risks are created and new problems can result. Similarly, as corrective actions accumulate over time, they can increase the complexity of a process or a product and increase the likelihood of failure. Consider the effects of inadequate actions or cumulative actions, and be willing to "unlearn" from experience.

Inadequate or Incomplete Analysis. Look for investigations that do not determine cause, investigations without proposed actions, proposed actions that are not implemented, and actions that are ineffective. Inadequate and incomplete analysis can signal business culture dominance and/or lack of adequate resources.

Lack of Potential Problem Analysis. Look for actions designed to prevent problems. Risk-based decision-making groups generally have two major agendas: solve known problems and anticipate or prevent potential problems.

If the group cannot find the time or the resources to consider potential problems, especially those directly related to known problems, then the corporation remains at risk. Preventing problems requires more than is usually required by regulators, but prevention can have the greatest impact on the safety:profit equation over time.

WHEN MANAGEMENT FAILS

Blaming management, especially in retrospective analysis of problems, is as shortsighted as frequent "employee error" citations in deviation records. Yes, management can be responsible for the ineffectiveness of the risk-based decision-making groups, but it is always more instructive to know how or why management fails.

When it appears that management has failed to respond effectively to a problem, consider that all information that reaches top management is censored, and that this censorship can be responsible for shortsighted or poor decision making. Three things contribute to this censorship: (a) Information flowing to top management is restricted to reduce information overload. (b) Specialization remains an obstacle to interpretation when information is highly technical in nature. (c) Uncertainty about understanding information, or knowing how it connects to product safety and performance, forces top decision makers to rely on *what they feel* or *think they know* rather than on *what they know*. (1) Audit the route of information flow to management for these potential weaknesses before they become barriers to problem solving.

THE EXTRA CHALLENGES OF INNOVATIVE TECHNOLOGIES

When risk taking is the nature of the business, as it is in new, innovative technologies and entrepreneurial ventures, it is very difficult to guard against the normalization of deviance (1) and to maintain a lasting distinction between the definition of acceptable risk vs. unacceptable risk.

In product development, deviation from specification is common, as one learns product and process capabilities. Similarly, rules are made, challenged, and then remade as more is learned. In this environment, risks are continuously reassessed and specifications changed. Once a product is authorized for distribution in the commercial market, however, this approach to change is unacceptable. This shift in culture, required when a start-up company moves from product development and clinical investigations into GMP/QSR manufacturing and testing, is difficult to make—especially when existing product developers are asked to wear two hats, one for innovative product development and the other for regulated manufacturing.

In addition, risks associated with new or innovative technologies can change with time and market experience. Radioactivity, once considered harmless, is now considered a high-risk hazard. One need only recall photographs of the first A-bomb explosions, with observers wearing sunglasses for protection, as an example:

> "As late as 1949, the director of the U.S. Navy's Ordnance Branch told a congressional committee that you could stand in the open at one end of the north-south runway at the Washington National Airport, with no more protection than the clothes you now have on, and have an atomic bomb explode at the other end of the runway without serious injury to you." (6)

Similarly, in recent years market launch has changed the risk analysis of bovine growth hormone use in milk cows, and genetically altered foods as well.

CITED REFERENCES

1. Vaughn, Diane. 1996. *The Challenger Launch Decision*. Chicago: University of Chicago Press.

2. Unseem, Michael. 1998. "Eugene Kranz Returns Apollo 13 to Earth," *The Leadership Moment*. New York: Times Books, Random House.

3. Langewiesche, William. 1998. "The Lessons of Valu-Jet 592." *Atlantic Monthly* (March).

4. Hammond, John S., Ralph L. Keeney, and Howard Raiffa. 1998. "The Hidden Traps in Decision Making." *Harvard Business Review* (September–October).

5. Zaleznik, Abraham. 1997. "Real Work." *Harvard Business Review* (November–December).

6. Sagan, Scott D. 1993. *Limits of Safety*. Princeton, NJ: Princeton University Press.

7. Krakauer, Jon. 1997. *Into Thin Air*. New York: Villard Books.

8. Linderman, Gerald F. 1997. "Discipline: Not the American Way," *World Within War*. New York: The Free Press.

9. Hampden-Turner, Charles, and Alfons Trompenaars. 1993. *The Seven Cultures of Capitalism*. New York: Doubleday.

10. Pool, Robert. 1997. *Beyond Engineering*. New York: Oxford University Press.

CHAPTER 9

ORGANIZATIONAL DESIGN: A NEW APPROACH

Eliminating, preventing, or minimizing the impact of accidents-of-design and accidents-of-procedure requires more than the well-integrated, risk-based decision-making processes presented in Section II. Eliminating, preventing, or minimizing the impact of accidents-of-management requires more than an awareness of potential socio-technical problems, presented in Section III. A successful, cost-effective, risk-based approach to product development and manufacturing also requires a new approach to organizational design. A new approach is needed because:

- The worker in this industry has two responsibilities. Primarily and traditionally, the worker performs a task as directed. Secondly, however, the worker is also a source of information about the performance of the products and their associated manufacturing and testing processes. Without an organizational structure that accommodates both a centralized approach to management to ensure that work is done as directed and a decentralized approach to management to ensure that the information required to prevent and solve problems is captured, the business of medical product development and manufacturing will suffer.
- Revised communication networks between management and worker will provide the requisite efficiencies mandated as a company moves from development to commercialization, or as a company downsizes in response to mergers and acquisitions.

- Managing a responsible, knowledgeable worker requires different skills than managing a subservient worker does, and a different management: worker relationship.

A New Organizational "Chart"

In the medical product industry, management is primarily responsible for developing and manufacturing products that are safe and effective for their intended use, and distributing those products to the intended users. The functional areas of the corporation that fulfill this mission are Development, Operations (Manufacturing and Testing), and Distribution. Without these functional areas, coordinated to work as efficiently and effectively as possible to produce acceptable product, the company will fail. These groups form the "productive core" of the company; all other functional areas support or protect this core. Consult Figure 9.1.

Development, manufacturing, testing, and distribution of products requires resources. These resources include money, materials, equipment, personnel, documents and standards, facility and utility systems, working environments, and customers. The functional areas of the corporation that acquire, qualify, and provide these resources include Purchasing, Materials Management, Maintenance Engineering, Quality Control, and Human Resources.

In addition, every company needs to protect its productive core from the effects of known hazards and unexpected events. This requires hazard identification, risk analysis, deviation monitoring, and responsible risk-based decision making to enable quick and effective responses to problems in operations or in the market. The functional areas that protect the "productive core" include Quality Assurance, Regulatory Affairs, Information Systems Management, Validation/Technical Services, and Customer Service.

An organizational model, illustrating this perspective, is provided in Figure 9.1. In this figure, the productive core of the company (Development > Operations > Distribution) is served and protected by Quality and Compliance Services that wrap around the core to serve and protect the productive core. Functional areas of Quality and Compliance Services that form the internal "service center" to coordinate and integrate activities between business units and troubleshoot problems include Materials Management, Maintenance Engineering, Document Management, Quality Control, Quality Assurance, and Validation. Functional areas of Quality and Compliance Services that form the external "protective layer" to provide liaisons between the company and other allied partners, regulators, customers or vendors include Regulatory Affairs, Record Management, Purchasing, Sales/Marketing, Customer Service, Legal, and Finance.

FIGURE 9.1
ORGANIZATIONAL DESIGN THAT SUPPORTS RISK MANAGEMENT

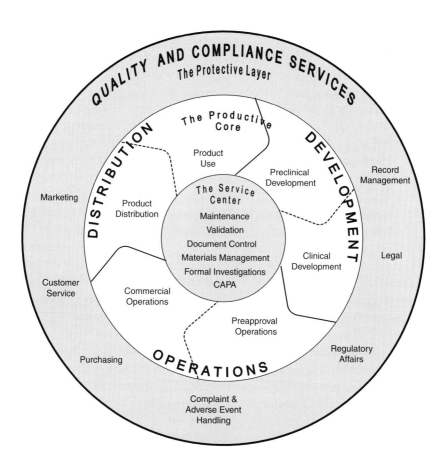

The organizational structure illustrated in Figure 9.1 differs significantly from the traditional, box-and-line organization charts. This is intentional. As suggested previously, management needs to reconsider the traditional approach to business in the medical products industry. Changing the visual image of the organizational chart can initiate essential change in management:worker relationships. (1)

PEOPLE-BASED VS. FUNCTION-BASED ORGANIZATIONAL DESIGNS

In start-up companies or newly acquired companies, organizational designs evolve over time, based on the personalities of key managers and executives. If a QC manager is hired that has QA experience, QA and QC are combined into one department; if a QA manager is hired that has regulatory experience, QA and Regulatory are combined into one department; if a Regulatory manager is hired that has clinical experience, Regulatory and Clinical Affairs are combined into one department. With limited resources, building a new company or a new division can encourage creative organizational design. Although a "people-based" organizational design can serve the start-up company for many years — or at least until product launch — it can cripple a growing organization with redundancies, inefficiencies, and lack of focused expertise if left in effect too long.

Similarly, in companies that have been the victim of mergers, acquisitions, and reallocation of personnel due to downsizing, organizational designs degrade over time. Management, challenged with limited resources and production pressures, reorganizes based on who can do what and who is willing to do what. Again, a people-based approach to organizational design dominates.

People-based organizational designs depend on individual performance; function-based organizations depend on systems. As a result, people-based organizations are vulnerable to the variability of performance and commitment from individuals; people make mistakes, quit, retire, or just lose interest. People-based organizational designs depend on individuals who "wear many hats"; function-based organizational designs create and encourage expertise. As a result, people-based organizations find recruitment and replacement of personnel difficult, as job descriptions contain uniquely diverse skill sets; and function-based organizations can more easily recruit expertise for common company functions.

Function-based organizational designs provide an essential flexibility in medical product manufacturing. Changes in regulations, technologies, and products can require changes in the allocation of resources and responsibilities. Only when these resources and responsibilities are defined along functional criteria, and only when the requirements of the functional units-of-operation are clearly defined, can a company respond to change quickly and in a cost-effective manner by reallocating responsibilities for predefined functional units-of-operation.

Establish Functional Units-of-Operation for the Organization

As discussed in Chapter 7, theorists emphasize that intelligent organizational design depends on a balance between centralized and decentralized authority. This balance relies on clearly defined roles and responsibilities and on well-trained, well-rehearsed management-workforce interactions. In an organization dedicated to this approach, the roles and responsibilities of functional areas must be defined either as components of the productive core or as quality and compliance services provided to the productive core. The roles and responsibilities must provide for both authority and responsibility in logically integrated and related tasks, and these roles and responsibilities should be established in controlled documents. Defining roles and responsibilities will:

- facilitate their assignment to specific functional areas
- minimize redundancies of effort when more than one group thinks it is responsible for a given task
- minimize neglect of responsibilities when more than one group is responsible and assume the other group has done the work
- provide compliance with quality system regulations for device and diagnostic companies (21 CFR 820.30).

Before standards of authority and responsibility can be written, the functional requirements of the organization need to be identified. First establish the purpose of the corporation. What are the products? What services does the company provide commercially? What is the market for these products and services (U.S., Europe, Japan, rest of world)? Does the company provide contract manufacturing services in addition to manufacturing its own products? Does the company develop its own products? What business units form the productive core of the company?

Tofte Medical, for example, develops, manufactures, and markets sterile, liquid drug products in glass vials. These products are distributed in the U.S. and Europe. The business unit components of their productive core are:

- Development
  - Research and Pre-Clinical Product Development
  - Clinical Product Development
- Operations
  - Preapproval Operations (Process Development, Scale-up, Validation)
  - Operations (Formulation, Sterilization, Filling/Stoppering, Capping, Inspection, Testing, Labeling, Packaging)

- Market Distribution

After the business units are identified, next identify the resources required to do this work.

Tofte Medical requires the following resources:
- People/Employees
- Equipment
- Materials and Processing Intermediates
- Facilities and/or Production and Testing Environments
- Utility Production Systems
- Customers
- Money
- Information: Documents, Instructions, Standards, Specifications

When products/services, business units, and resources are identified, designate logical, separable, functional units-of-operation. Although it is convenient to think of units-of-operation in terms of existing or standard functional areas, it is recommended that the list be developed as stand-alone responsibilities. Consider and include the functional units-of-operation/responsibility identified in the QSRs, GMPs, and ISO 9001 documents. The ultimate goal of identifying separable, functional units-of-operation is to reassemble them into logical Quality System Components (QSCs) for the corporation. See Exhibit 9.1 for an example of QSCs and functional units-of-operation.

Establish Roles and Responsibilities for Functional Units-of-Operation

Establish functional units-of-operation in Quality System Component (QSC) commitment documents; for an example consult Exhibits 9.3 and 9.4. These types of documents provide a mechanism for executive management to communicate its expectations for compliance with laws, regulations, industry guidelines, and company standards to the next level of management. In turn, these same documents provide a mechanism for middle management to outline and connect these commitments to routine operations. QSC documents establish company standards and practices that:
- assure the continuing quality of resources, processes, and products over time
- provide a road map to an interacting set of protocols, programs, and procedures that fulfill commitments
- assign responsibility for the management of a functional unit-of-operation
- assure harmonization between sites or divisions of a corporation.

Each QSC document is owned by a functional area. Management in the functional area is responsible for assuring that the commitments made in a

QSC are fulfilled and that information is collected, on a continuing basis, as evidence of compliance. Format and content guidance for a QSC document is provided in Exhibit 9.2; example QSC documents are in Exhibits 9.3 and 9.4. In companies that are required to have a Quality Manual, the QSC documents can be assembled as the major components of the manual.

Designate Authority and Responsibility

QSC documents assign responsibility; the authority to do the work referenced in the QSC, however, can be delegated to other functional areas. One can delegate the authority but not the responsibility for quality in a function-based organization. In other words, not all tasks or duties identified in a QSC are fulfilled by one functional area.

Preventive maintenance (PM) and calibration of equipment, for example, are the responsibility of the Maintenance/Engineering (M/E) department at Tofte Medical. This means that M/E is responsible for the PM and calibration of *all* equipment in the facility, including laboratory equipment. Traditionally, however, laboratory equipment has been maintained and calibrated by QC. In the QSC of a function-based organization, this does *not* need to change. The responsibility for PM/calibration of laboratory equipment belongs to M/E, but the authority of the work can remain in QC. In routine practice, schedules for laboratory equipment PM/calibration are maintained in M/E and issued to QC on a monthly basis. When PM and calibration are completed by QC, a report is provided to M/E.

Managing the Responsible Worker

The key resource of the corporation in traditional, low-tech industries is money, and success depends on attracting and holding the company's financiers. The key resource of the corporation in high-tech industries, however, is the worker, and success depends on attracting, holding, and motivating these individuals. The high-tech worker is a partner in the business, and management practices must recognize and facilitate their involvement. (2)

As mentioned previously, companies that rely on efficient problem solving to maintain profitability require consistent, decentralized decision-making from all employees. In this scenario management relies on a worker to follow directions and to provide feedback information on the outcome of the task and/or the adequacy of the instructions. Management, as a result, must be able to direct the worker and be directed by the worker. Managers must learn to coordinate and support rather than control the worker.

Profitable manufacturing of safe medical products requires planning and vigilance. Management is responsible for planning and management is responsible for creating an environment in which workers are vigilant. When worker input is valued and used routinely in risk-based decision making, product safety and production efficiencies improve over time.

CITED REFERENCES

1. Hampden-Turner, Charles, and Alfons Trompenaars. 1993. "On Synchrony, Hierarchy and Time," *The Seven Cultures of Capitalism*. New York: A Currency Book by Doubleday.

2. Drucker, Peter. 1999. "Beyond the Information Revolution." *Atlantic Monthly* (October), pp. 47–57.

Exhibit 9.1

Page __1__ of __3__

Business Units, Quality System Components, and Functional Units-of-Operation

In the listing that follows, Business Units are indicated in bold, caps, Quality System Components are indicated with (•), and Functional units-of-operation are indicated as (–).

DEVELOPMENT
- • Design Control
  - – Pre-clinical development and verification
  - – Clinical design validation
  - – Design and process change
- • Specification Control
  - – Final product specifications and/or device master records
  - – Materials, components, labeling, reagents, standards
  - – Equipment and equipment systems
  - – Testing processes
  - – Manufacturing processes

OPERATIONS
- • Production Control/Scheduling
- • Process Control and Qualification/Validation
  - – Identification and status labeling of materials/product in area
  - – Component preparation
  - – Equipment preparation
  - – Product area preparation
  - – Formulation/subassembly preparation
  - – Sterilization
  - – Inspection
  - – Labeling
  - – Packaging
  - – Transfer of materials within manufacturing area
- • Testing Control/Scheduling
- • Analytical Test Method Control and Qualification/Validation
  - – Identification and status labeling of samples in area
  - – Chemical testing
  - – Biological testing
  - – Physical testing
  - – Microbiological testing
  - – Data management and notification
  - – Transfer of materials within area
  - – Product distribution and control

Exhibit 9.1 (continued)

Page 2 of 3

Business Units, Quality System Components and Functional Units-of-Operation

PRODUCT CONTROL
- Regulatory Control
  - Notifications
  - Applications for approval and change
- Product disposition management
- Product stability monitoring system
- Marketing control
  - Post-market surveillance
  - Customer service

RESOURCE MANAGEMENT AND CONTROL
- Material and Product Management and Control
  - Purchasing of materials
  - Receiving of materials and intermediates
  - Identification, control, and status labeling of materials/products
  - Material dispositioning
  - Inventory control of materials and product
  - Warehouse control
  - Materials/product transfer control
  - Processing intermediates and test sample shipping control
  - Returned goods control
  - Vendor/supplier identification, qualification, contracts, and monitoring
- Information/Data Management
  - Document control
  - Record control
  - Data control
  - Statistical control
  - Software control and qualification
  - Vendor identification, qualification, contracts, and monitoring
- Personnel Management and Control
  - Organization and functional areas of responsibility
  - Personnel recruitment and hiring
  - Personnel training and development
  - Personnel performance assessments
  - Contractors/consultants: identification, qualification, contracts, and monitoring
- Equipment Management and Control
  - Equipment specifications/performance standards
  - Equipment purchasing

Exhibit 9.1 (continued)

Page __3__ of __3__

Business Units, Quality System Components and Functional Units-of-Operation

- Equipment installation and qualification
- Equipment performance monitoring
- Preventive maintenance
- Equipment calibration
- Equipment repair
- Utility Production System Management
  - Water for injection production and distribution system control
  - Purified water production and distribution system control
  - Clean steam production and distribution system control
  - HVAC system production and distribution control
  - Compressed air production and distribution system control
  - Fire prevention and control systems
  - Waste collection and treatment system control
  - Cooling systems control
- Environmental Control/Contamination Control Qualification and Monitoring
  - Clean rooms
  - Controlled production areas
  - Specialized equipment environments (incubators, hoods, storage chambers)
  - Environmental monitoring contractors: identification, qualification, contracts, and monitoring
- Building/Facility Control
  - Design: layout/flow of materials, personnel, product, waste, air
  - Grounds and exterior building maintenance
  - Cleaning and contamination control in general support areas
  - Waste removal
  - Equipment location
  - Pest and insect control
  - Building security
  - Contractor identification, qualification, contracts and monitoring
  - Safety standards, control and monitoring: physical, chemical, biological, radiation

RISK MANAGEMENT AND CONTROL

- Data of Exception, Monitoring, Investigation and Action Identification (Complaints, OOSRs, Deviations, Audit Observations)
- Data of Compliance, Auditing/Monitoring, Trending, and Action Proposals
- Corrective and Preventive Action Implementation and Follow-up
- Management Control of Partnerships or Business Liaison for Development, Operations, and Distribution: Identification, Qualification, Contracts, and Monitoring

Exhibit 9.2

Page __1__ of __1__

Quality System Component Documents: Format and Content Guidelines

Title: Quality System Component

1.0 Purpose/Scope
Briefly describe the section or component of the Quality System that is covered by the commitments and requirements of this document. Use terminology or reference the terminology that is commonly used to describe these systems in corporate documents. Designate the corporate divisions, sites, product lines, and/or functional areas of the corporation that are within the scope of this document.

2.0 System Commitments and Requirements
Designate the commitments or requirements of this Quality System Component in general terms. These commitments should be fulfilled by procedures and practices of the corporation. They should be commitments that apply across product lines and often across multiple sites of operation.

3.0 Commitment Owner and Functional Area
Indicate which functional area(s) is responsible for fulfilling the commitments of the QSC.

4.0 References
List all references that are considered relevant to the specified quality system component. List all appropriate CFR citations and any guideline documents from FDA or EU. When dates are omitted from a citation, it will be assumed that the citation refers to the most current version of the document.

5.0 Definitions
Define any terms used in the Quality System Component document or any terms likely to be used extensively in the documents that support this quality system component.

6.0 System Design Features and Processes
This section of the Quality System Component document should be organized to present the major features, processes, and flow that are required to support or fulfill the commitment and requirements listed in section 2.0. For each specific commitment listed in section 2.0, either describe how that commitment will be fulfilled or refer to another lower-level document (procedure, specification, protocol, etc.) that provides this description. All commitments must be supported, meaning that there are or will be working documents in place to describe how the commitments will be fulfilled.

Exhibit 9.3

Page __1__ of __3__

Example Quality System Component Document

Title: Material and Product Control and Management System

1.0 Purpose/Scope
This document establishes corporate commitments for managing materials and products at the Tofte, MN facility. Commitments include purchasing, receipt, inspection/test, identification, storage, inventory control, movement, and use of materials, as well as commitments for the identification, storage, inventory control, shipment and tracking of products.

2.0 System Commitments and Requirements
Commitments to material and product management include:
- All items purchased for use in the production and testing of products are purchased from vendors that have successfully completed a vendor qualification process.
- All services contracted to support the production, testing, and distribution of products are contracted from organizations that have been evaluated and found acceptable to provide such services.
- All materials, components, labels, reagents, etc., used in the production and testing of products are completely identified with part numbers, control numbers (lot numbers), and status indicators (released for use).
- All materials received into the facility are recorded and evaluated (inspected/tested) to assure that they meet preestablished specifications for quality.
- Movement of materials and product within the facility and to/from outside contractors is controlled (documented).
- All product in the facility, in all stages of production, is identified completely (part numbers, lot numbers, and status indicators), and products are segregated in storage based on status (quarantine, released or nonconforming/rejected).
- Warehousing practices to assure:
  - clean, orderly, and secure storage conditions
  - controlled and appropriate environmental conditions of storage
  - segregated storage of materials/products in different stages of manufacture
  - segregated storage of materials/products of differing status
  - inventory control systems for materials and products.
- All product distribution is conducted in a manner that assures a record of accountability and traceability.
- Product returns are controlled to prevent mix-up with product for distribution.
- Records that provide evidence for ongoing control/management of materials and product are retained, e.g., inventory control records, product distribution records, scheduling records, specification testing records, warehouse cleaning records, and environmental control records.

Exhibit 9.3 (continued)

Page __2__ of __3__

Example Quality System Component Document

3.0 Commitment Owner and Functional Area
Materials Management is responsible for the design and implementation of the materials/product management system presented in this document and for establishing associated procedures.

4.0 References
- 21 CFR 820.50 (a)   Purchasing Control: Evaluation of Suppliers
- 21 CFR 820.50 (b)   Purchasing Control: Purchasing Data
- 21 CFR 820.60   Identification of Product
- 21 CFR 820.65   Traceability of Product
- 21 CFR 820.70 (h)   Production & Process Control: Manufacturing Material
- 21 CFR 820.80 (b)   Receiving Acceptance Activities
- 21 CFR 820.90   Nonconforming Product
- 21 CFR 820.120 (b) Labeling Inspection
- 21 CFR 820.120 (c) Labeling Storage
- 21 CFR 820.140   Handling
- 21 CFR 820.150   Storage
- 21 CFR 820.160   Distribution
- 21 CFR 211.80   Control of Components: General Requirements
- 21 CFR 211.82   Receipt and Storage of Untested . . .
- 21 CFR 211.86   Use of Approved Components . . .
- 21 CFR 211.89   Rejected Components
- 21 CFR 211.142   Warehousing Practices
- 21 CFR 211.150   Distribution Procedures
- 21 CFR 211.184   Component, Container, Closure, & Labeling Records
- 21 CFR 211.204   Returned Drug Product
- ISO 9001/EN46001   4.3 Contract Review
- ISO 9001/EN46001   4.6 Purchasing
- ISO 9001/EN46001   4.8 Product ID and Traceability
- ISO 9001/EN46001   4.10 Inspection and Test
- ISO 9001/EN46001   4.12 Inspection and Test Status
- ISO 9001/EN46001   4.13 Control of Nonconforming product
- ISO 9001/EN46001   4.15 Handling, Storage, and Delivery
- ISO 13485: 4.6.3   Purchasing Controls
- ISO 13485: 4.8 a,b Product Identification and Traceability
- ISO 13485: 4.15   Packing, Storage, Delivery

Exhibit 9.3 (continued)

Page __3__ of __3__

Example Quality System Component Document

5.0 Definitions
Materials — components, chemicals, subassemblies, printed materials that are used to manufacture products

Products — product that is available for commercial distribution

6.0 System Design Features and Processes

6.1 Purchasing Controls
See SOP MT002

6.2 Production Planning/Scheduling
See SOP MT011

6.3 Receipt of Incoming Materials
See SOP MT009

6.4 Identification and Inspection/Test of Incoming Materials
See SOP MT008

6.5 Movement of Materials
See SOP MT003

6.6 Material/Product Storage Practices
See SOP MT004

6.7 Product Identification and Traceability
See SOP MT005

6.8 Distribution of Final Product
See SOP MT006

6.9 Shipment/Receipt of Production Intermediates and Test Samples
See SOP MT007

6.10 Supplier/Vendor Qualification and Monitoring
See SOP QA002

6.11 Returned Goods Procedures
See SOP MT311

Exhibit 9.4

Page __1__ of __3__

Example Quality System Component Document

Title: Production Control and Management System

1.0 Purpose/Scope

This document establishes the commitments for managing the production of products, components, and intermediates at Tofte Medical and its contractors.

2.0 System Commitments and Requirements

Commitments to production control include:
- planning and/or scheduling of production events
- staging each production event in a manner that ensures complete identification and control of resources, i.e.,
  - production event preclearance to occur before the work begins
  - use of processes for production, established in DMR and procedures, that have been reviewed and approved for use and/or validated
  - controlled issue of production documents for use on a lot-by-lot basis for SWB products
  - controlled use of materials as directed by DMR and SOPs
  - controlled use of equipment as directed by DMR and SOPs
  - maintenance of and controlled use of manufacturing locations/environments
  - use of trained production personnel
  - identification and status labeling of all in-process and final product in production area
  - identification of activities within production area while activities are in progress (room status identifiers)
- evidence of compliance with controls, available on a lot-by-lot basis, as manufacturing records, forms, log-books
- complete accountability (reconciliation) of components and materials
- a commitment to control and evaluate any changes to processes
- a commitment to investigate any observations of out-of-specification results from in-process testing, yield failures, or reconciliation failures

3.0 Commitment Owner and Functional Area

Manufacturing is responsible for the design and implementation of the production management system and for establishing associated procedures for these systems.

Exhibit 9.4 (continued)

Page __2__ of __3__

Example Quality System Component Document

4.0 References
- 21 CFR 820.70 (a)   Production and Process Controls: General
- 21 CFR 820.70 (b)   Production and Process Controls: Changes
- 21 CFR 820.70 (c)   Production and Process Controls: Environmental
- 21 CFR 820.70 (e)   Production and Process Controls: Contamination
- 21 CFR 820.80 (c)   In-process Acceptance Activities
- 21 CFR 820.90 (b,2)   Nonconformity Review and Disposition/Rework
- 21 CFR 820.120 (a)   Device Labeling: Label Integrity
- 21 CFR 820.120 (b)   Device Labeling: Label Inspection
- 21 CFR 820.120 (d)   Device Labeling: Labeling Operations
- 21 CFR 820.120 (e)   Device Labeling: Control Number
- 21 CFR 820.130   Device Packing
- 21 CFR 211.100   Production/Process Control: Procedures
- 21 CFR 211.101   Production/Process Control: Charge-in Components
- 21 CFR 211.103   Production/Process Control: Calculation of Yield
- 21 CFR 211.105   Production/Process Control: Equipment Identification
- 21 CFR 211.111   Production/Process Control: Time Limits
- 21 CFR 211.113   Production/Process Control: Contamination Control
- 21 CFR 211.115   Production/Process Control: Reprocessing
- 21 CFR 211.122   Packaging/Labeling Control: Materials Exam/Use
- 21 CFR 211.125   Packaging/Labeling Control: Labeling Issuance
- 21 CFR 211.130   Packaging/Labeling Control: Operations
- 21 CFR 211.186   Master Production and Control Records
- 21 CFR 211.188   Batch Production and Control Records
- ISO 9001/EN46001:4.9   Process Control
- ISO 13485: 4.9   Process Control
- ISO 13485: 4.10.3   In–Process Inspection and Test
- ISO 13485: 4.13.2   Nonconforming Product
- ISO 13485: 4.15   Packing, Handling, Storage, Delivery

5.0 Definitions
Production – processes include assembly, formulation, packaging, inspection, labeling, and holding in storage.

Exhibit 9.4 (continued)

Page __3__ of __3__

Example Quality System Component Document

6.0 System Design Features and Processes

6.1 Product-Specific Flow Diagrams
See SOP PR566

6.2 Production Area Identification and Use
See SOP PR421

6.3 Production Area Cleaning and Disinfection
See SOP PR423

6.4. Production Staging and Preclearance
See SOP PR398

6.5 In-process Monitoring of Production Parameters
See SOP PR222

6.6 Process Change
See SOP QA034

6.7 Manufacturing Record Management
See SOP QA112

6.8 Product Identification and Status
See SOP MT217

Glossary

Acceptable risk – risk that is reduced to a level that is determined to be acceptable, given the probability that a failure will occur and lead to a clinical effect and given the severity of its impact.

Accidents-of-design – material, process, and product failures that should be predicted and eliminated or prevented during design and validation but are not.

Accidents-of-management – accidents that result from an environment in which poor decision making occurs for a variety of reasons.

Accidents-of-procedure – accidents that occur because mistakes occur during product use or during the performance of a manufacturing or testing process.

Action Analysis Team – a group of individuals that provides the business perspective to the actions proposed by the Formal Investigation Team.

Action implementation planning protocol – a document that identifies (a) resources and procedures required to implement corrective or preventive actions, (b) monitoring requirements to determine the effectiveness of actions, and (c) acceptance criteria for the testing or observations associated with monitoring.

Action levels – a range of values between alert levels and specifications that, when exceeded, signal an apparent drift from normal operating conditions. When the action level range is reached, action is required.

Adverse event – any unfavorable or unintended medical occurrence in a patient or subject associated with the use of a medical product, whether or not it is considered related to the medical product.

AIPP – see action implementation planning protocols.

Alert levels – a range of values that, when exceeded, signal a potential drift from normal operating conditions. Alert level ranges fall between normal operating ranges and action level ranges.

CCP – see critical control point.

Complaint – any written, electronic, or oral communication that alleges deficiencies related to the identity, quality, durability, reliability, safety, effectiveness, or performance of a product, after it has been released for distribution.

Critical control point – a step in processing at which control can be applied and that is critical in the prevention or elimination of a product safety hazard or in its reduction to an acceptable level.

Critical process – a manufacturing process that creates a critical product attribute, or a testing process that determines if a product has met a critical product attribute specification.

Critical product attribute – a product attribute that contributes to the safety of a product, in that the lack of the attribute or variation in its control would adversely affect product safety for the patient or customer/user.

Culture of blame – a working environment in which employees are routinely blamed for accidents and problems; the resulting secrecy in this working environment inhibits the ability to improve operations and product performance.

Culture of responsibility – a working environment in which employees are informed and responsible for reporting problems and making observations about products and processes that can be used to improve operations and product performance.

Data-of-compliance observation – information or data that meets specifications and/or established standards of practice.

Data-of-exception observation – information or data that does not meet specifications and/or established standards of practice, including deviations, discrepancies, nonconforming units, alert limits, action limits, and invalid test results.

Design validation – demonstrating that a product performs as intended in the user environment, in the hands of the intended user; e.g., clinical studies.

Direct action implementation – actions that can be implemented without conducting a formal investigation.

ECP – see essential control point.

Essential control point – Process control point that, although not directly related to product safety, is nevertheless essential for process reliability and effectiveness in that deviation from processing limits or acceptance criteria would seriously compromise the reliability or effectiveness of the process.

Failure mode effects and criticality analysis – a standard procedure (e.g., U.S. Military Standard MIL-STD 1629A) in which each potential failure mode in a product is analyzed to determine the results or effects on the product and to classify each failure mode according to its severity; this is a bottom-up approach to risk analysis.

FMECA – see failure mode effects and criticality analysis.

Formal Investigation – a systematic process of information gathering and analysis conducted to identify the cause of a problem or unexpected observation.

Function-based organizational design – an organizational design that designates job responsibilities based on the functional requirements of the organization.

HACCP – see hazard analysis and critical control point.

Hazard analysis and critical control point – a systematic approach to the identification, evaluation and control of process controls that control product safety hazards. The principles and applications of HACCP were developed in 1997 by the U.S. FDA, Department of Agriculture, and the National Advisory Committee on Microbiological Criteria for Foods to provide a format for process control point identification and evaluation. The guideline was created to help food processors and distributors ensure that foods are safe for consumption by providing an effective and rational means of assuring food safety from harvest to consumption.

Harm – physical injury and/or damage to the health of people, property, or the environment.

Hazard – a potential source of harm.

High reliability theory – a theory that maintains that intelligent organizational design and management techniques in a company can compensate for individual weaknesses within the organization and assure accident-free operations. Theorists believe that there are four critical, causal factors that produce positive safety records within a wide variety of organizations: leadership that prioritizes safety objectives as a corporate goal, high levels of redundancy for product safety and essential personnel, a corporate culture of high reliability at the line level that is well rehearsed, and a rigorous, organizational approach to trial-and-error learning.

High-risk hazard – a hazard likely to cause serious harm and likely to occur.

Information monitoring programs – procedures that direct the collection of data and observations about the performance of products and processes over time, e.g., environmental monitoring programs, adverse event monitoring of product performance, etc.

Level I observation – an unexpected result or deviation that is not likely to affect the performance or safety of the product.

Level II observation – an unexpected result or deviation that has the potential to significantly affect product performance or manufacturing/testing process performance.

Level III observation – an unexpected result or deviation that has potential serious impact on the safety of the product *and* the product is in the market or the clinic, i.e., an Adverse Event.

Market withdrawal – removal or correction of a distributed product because of a minor violation that would not be subject to legal action by FDA, e.g., normal stock rotation practices, routine equipment adjustments and repair.

Nonreportable event – an event that is not reportable; see reportable event.

Normal accident theory – these theorists maintains that, even with intelligent organizational design and management techniques in a company, as suggested by the high-reliability theorists, serious accidents are inevitable.

Normalization of deviance – the process by which groups of people can learn to accept deviant observations as normal because of a variety of environmental influences.

Out-of-specification result – an observation or test result that does not meet predetermined expectations or specifications.

PCP – see process control point.

People-based organizational design – an organizational design that is developed from the individual capabilities of the employees rather than the functional requirements of the organization.

Preliminary evaluation – an evaluation conducted as soon as possible after an event or observation made in the market is known to the company to confirm the observation and triage the observation for appropriate action.

Preliminary investigation – an investigation conducted at or near the point of the unexpected result or observation, by the observer and/or a supervisor, and as soon as possible after the event has been recorded or observed to confirm the observation and triage the observation for appropriate action.

Probability of occurrence – the likelihood that, despite mitigating factors, the cause of a potential hazard will occur and lead to an identified failure mode and result in an Adverse Event.

Process control point – the steps in processing where biological, chemical, or physical factors are controlled, in order to provide greater assurance that a process will perform reliably.

Process validation – demonstrating that a process performs as intended, in the environment of routine use.

Product requirements – requirements that describe a product's intended purpose, and all safety and effectiveness characteristics that the product must possess to achieve its intended purpose. These are also called design input requirements by FDA.

Product risk analysis – the use of available information to identify all hazards associated with product use and estimate the risks to which the product users and the environment of use are exposed during product use.

Product risk analysis report – a document that provides the results of risk analysis for a particular product. Risks associated with product features and attributes are identified and risk levels designated, such as high, medium, or low risk.

Product specification document – a document that establishes the product specifications.

Recall – removal or correction of a marketed product, by a company, that regulatory authorities consider to be in violation of the laws they administer and against which regulatory authorities would initiate legal action.

Reportable event – an event that requires a manufacturer, distributor, or user to file a report with regulatory authorities; an event that reasonably suggests that a product has or may have caused or contributed to a death, serious injury, or malfunctioned and if the malfunction recurs it is likely to lead to serious injury or death.

Resources – the materials, information, equipment, environments, people and infrastructure essential to the implementation of an organization's policies and the achievement of its objectives.

Residual risk – risks remaining after protective measures have been taken.

Risk – a value based on combining the probability that harm will occur combined with the severity of that harm.

Risk, business – risks that affect the ability of the business to grow and prosper.

Risk, technical – risks that affect product safety/performance or development/manufacturing/testing process performance.

Risk analysis – the use of available information to identify hazards and to estimate risk.

Risk assessment – the overall process of risk analysis and risk evaluation.

Risk level matrix – a table that distinguishes acceptable risks from unacceptable risks by relating the severity of an effect-of-failure to the probability that the failure will occur.

Risk management – the systematic application of management policy, procedures, and practices to the tasks of analyzing, evaluating, and controlling risk.

Risk reduction – taking protective measures to reduce risk.

Risk-based decision making – a decision-making process that requires the consideration of risks associated with the outcome actions of the decision.

Risk-based decision-making groups – a group or team of individuals that is responsible for making risk-based decisions.

Serious adverse events – any adverse events associated with the use of the product that result in death, life-threatening illness, permanent disability, in-patient hospitalization or continued hospitalization, congenital anomaly, or required intervention to prevent permanent impairment.

Severity – a measure of the possible consequences of a hazard.

Specifications – a range of values associated with operational attributes, characteristics, or parameters beyond which the process, product, equipment system, support utility (water, steam, air, gas), or environment, etc., is considered unacceptable for use.

Triage – a process in which events, problems, actions, or items are sorted and work allocated based on priorities designed to maximize the benefits of the work.

Unacceptable risk – risk that is *not* acceptable, given the probability that a failure will occur and lead to a clinical effect and given the severity of its impact.

INDEX

accident theories, 2, 92-96
accidents-of-design, 2, 3, 19, 25-26, 89-92, 100, 119
accidents-of-management, 2-4, 25-26, 89-92, 96, 119
accidents-of-procedure, 2, 3, 19, 25-26, 89-92, 100, 119
action analysis and authorization, 69-71, 76-77
Action Analysis Team, 70, 78, 81-86, 101-118
action effectiveness assessments, 72, 81-86
Action Implementation Planning Protocols, 36, 57, 82-86
action implementation, 36, 57, 71-73, 77-78, 81-86
action limits, 35, 43, 45, 48
action review record, 78
Adverse Events, 36, 40, 51-62, 64, 66, 107, 121
alert limits, 35, 43, 45, 46, 48
bottom-up risk analysis, 12-13, 15, 22-23
business culture dominance, 103
business risk, 102-118
CAPA, 64, 120
complaints, 17-18, 36, 40, 51-59, 64, 107, 121
corrections and removals, 84
corrective action, 8, 17, 26, 85, 89, 96, 104
Critical Control Points, 26-33, 40, 67, 71, 84
critical process hazard analysis, 28-29
culture of responsibility, 38, 113-114, 125
culture of blame, 113-114
data-of-compliance trending, 44
data-of-compliance observations, 35-44, 52, 56, 58
data-of-exception observations, 35-44, 52, 55-59, 61-62, 64, 72

decentralized authority, 93, 95, 111, 114-115, 119
decision making rules, 111-112
Design Control, 18
Design Review Team, 96, 101-118
direct action implementation, 36, 41, 54, 57, 71, 82-83
environmental monitoring program, 47-49
Errors and Accidents, 40, 84
Essential Control Points, 29-30, 40-41, 71
failure mode, 13-14, 19, 23
Field Alerts, 40, 84
Formal Investigation team, 41, 44, 54, 56, 64-73, 101-118
Formal Investigation, 36, 40, 52, 55-58, 63-77, 81-86, 96
function-based organizational design, 122-123
group meeting controls, 64-65, 109-112
HACCP, 26-27
hazard analysis, 28-29
hazard identification, 10, 12-13
High Reliability theory, 92-96
information analysis, 68-71, 111, 116
information gathering, 54, 66-68, 74, 97-98
information monitoring program development, 41-43
information monitoring programs, 35-44, 47-49, 51-59
information quality, 110
information reporting variables, 97-98
ISO, 19, 26, 63, 116, 124
leadership, 93, 95, 101, 109, 112-118
levels of concern, 36, 40, 41, 44-46, 52, 54-58, 61-67, 70-71, 82, 84
Normal Accident theory, 93-96
normal operating conditions, 43
normalization of deviance, 96-97, 107-108
organizational design, 119-129
out-of-specification results, 8, 17, 35-36, 40, 41, 44-46, 52, 54-58, 61-62, 64, 75
overconfidence, 98-99, 109, 115
people-based organizational design, 122-123
post market feedback, 51-62
Preliminary Evaluation, 36, 52, 54, 55-57
Preliminary Investigations, 36, 39, 41, 44, 63, 64, 67, 72
probability ranking, 10-16, 22
process control points, 26-32

process deviations, 26, 31-32
process hazard analysis, 8, 25-30
process validation, 8, 17, 25, 30-31
product design verification/validation, 15, 18, 21, 23
product lifecycle, 8
Product Risk Analysis Reports, 8-9, 16-18, 37, 58
product risk analysis, 7-23, 58
productive core, 120-121, 123
profit vs. safety , 3, 59, 100, 125
Quality Manual, 125
quality system components, 124-125, 127-136
recalls, 84
redundancy, 93, 95
regulatory review, 36, 66, 71, 75, 77, 79, 82
reportable events, 56-58
reporting systems, FDA, 53
retrospective risk analysis, 18-19
risk analysis terminology, 7
risk analysis updates, 59
risk-based decision-making groups, 64-65, 70, 96-98, 101-118
risk benefit analysis, 16
risk level assignment, 13, 15
risk level matrix, 10-11, 15, 22
risk management framework, 36-37, 84
risk minimization, 13, 16
Serious Adverse Events, 53-62
severity ranking, 10-13, 15-17, 21
specifications , 15, 43, 45, 46
summit fever, 98-99, 109, 115
technical risk, 102-118
top-down risk analysis, 12-13, 15, 21
training, 43-44, 93-95, 102, 104-109, 110, 114
trending, 44, 58, 116
triage, 26, 40, 44, 46, 55-57, 66, 67, 73, 75, 106
trial and error learning, 94-95
units of operation, 123-124, 127-129